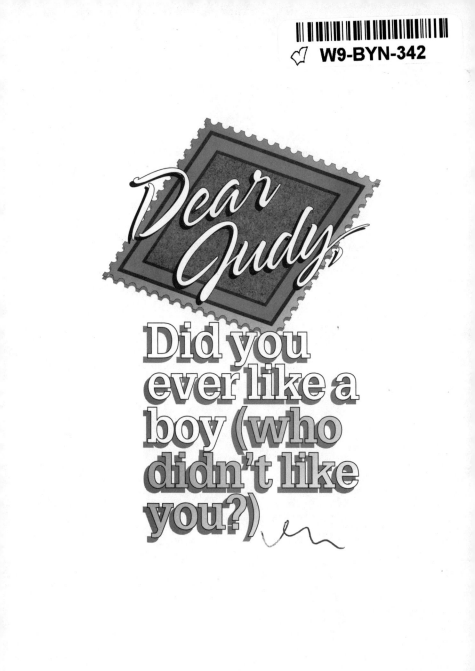

Dear Judy,

Did you ever like a boy (who didn't like you?)

Dear Judy,

Did you ever like a boy (who didn't like you?)

JUDY BAER

BETHANY HOUSE PUBLISHERS
Minneapolis, Minnesota 55438

Published by Bethany House Publishers
A Ministry of Bethany Fellowship, Inc.
11300 Hampshire Avenue South
Minneapolis, Minnesota 55438

Printed in the United States of America

Library of Congress Cataloging-in-Publication Data

Baer, Judy.
    Dear Judy, did you ever like a boy (who didn't like you?) / Judy Baer.
        p. cm.
    1. Teenage—United States—Juvenile literature. 2. Teenage girls—United States—Religious life—Juvenile literature. 3. Sex instruction for girls—United States. 4. Sex instruction for teenagers—United States. [1. Teenage girls. 2. Interpersonal relations. 3. Conduct of life. 4. Christian life.] I. Title.
HQ798.B28   1993
305.23'5—dc20   93–5940
ISBN 1–55661–341–5   CIP

JUDY BAER received a B.A. in English and Education from Concordia College in Moorhead, Minnesota. She has had over thirty novels published and is a member of the National Romance Writers of America, the Society of Children's Book Writers, and the National Federation of Press Women.

Two of her novels, *Adrienne* and *Paige*, have been prize-winning bestsellers in the Bethany House SPRING-FLOWER SERIES (for girls 12–15). Both books have been awarded first place for juvenile fiction in the National Federation of Press Women's communications contest.

RESPONSES TO THE CEDAR RIVER DAYDREAM SERIES

I like your books because I want to know what it's like being a teenager. I also need to know if it's really easy or hard to stay close to God.

—Georgina

You described my feelings exactly in your book New Girl in Town *even though I didn't move or have a retarded brother (but he IS very weird).*

—Dusty

These books have made me stronger in my faith. Thank you for that.

—Trudy

Your books are very helpful. Two days after I finished reading your first book, I had a similar problem to the one in the story. I remembered what Lexi did and handled my problem the same way. Everything worked out fine. I'm glad I had your book to relate to.

—Abby

Your books are great! They are true-to-life situations and each one focuses on problems that teens experience. It is a big help to read how Christian teens get through the tough times in life. These books help you take the pressure you get from your peers and use it constructively.

—Betty

CONTENTS

PART III: Faith and Friends

INTRODUCTION

What are the most frequently asked questions and most often expressed concerns that I receive from readers?

That's easy—they are questions about *friendship* (how to make friends and keep them) and about *boys*. These concerns are universal and, according to my readers, cause more hassles than any other part of teenage life. Friends and boys (which, hopefully, are not two entirely separate categories) are sources of both great pain and great pleasure. When you're having trouble with a friend, life can seem pretty bleak. If you're feeling popular and well liked the world looks sunny and bright.

But people—especially teenagers—can be fickle. You may be popular one day and an outcast the next. A great-looking boy might pay attention to you during class and then not recognize you in the hallway after school. Your best friend may suddenly refuse to speak to you or find a new BFF (that's Best Friend Forever!). How do you handle these and other problems? That's what this book is all about!

I've also discovered that you, my readers, identify very strongly with Lexi Leighton, a main character in the *Cedar River Daydreams* series. You've shared her pain in moving to a new place and making new friends (as in *New Girl in Town*) or boy trouble (as in *Yesterday's Dream*). Lexi is the character readers feel is most like them.

Why do you identify with Lexi? Probably because she is the kind of person you'd like to be. She tries to be a good and loyal friend (and does a credible job of it most of the time). Her motives are honest and loving. She attempts to live up to her ideals, to be popular, to do the right thing. My readers are terrific people who are doing the best they can—just like Lexi. See for yourself . . .

I have been reading your Cedar River Daydreams. I enjoy them very much. I feel as though I am right there with Lexi and her friends. Your writing makes me feel good. Although Lexi is older than me, I feel that we are alike.

—Polly, age 11

Where did you get your ideas for the series? Lexi reminds me of myself!

—Dora, age 12

You seem to know what interests teens. I can tell by the characters and topics you write about. In a lot of ways I am like Lexi. I look to her as an example. She has qualities and habits I would like to have. She is put in situations with friends that are very realistic.

—Morgan

Lexi Leighton has problems that I've had. After reading your books, I found it was easier to solve my problem.

—Farrah

I feel like Lexi is my firend. Sometimes I get into the stories so much I think they're real and not just a book.

—Ginger

I think its cool that all these things happen to Lexi and her friends. I feel for them. Your books are not fantasy. The stories are about real life. These things might actually happen to me. Lexi is like one of my friends.

—Sara

As Christian teenagers, you spend a lot of time in school, with your friends, moving about in the fascinating world God has created. You need to know how to live your faith without having to hide or separate yourself from the world in which you live. It is important that you know how to apply your beliefs to your life.

God should not be a remote friend that you visit only on Sundays. He should be an active, vital participant in every aspect of your life. He is interested in everything important to you—what happens to you on a date or if you're struggling with shyness or a tendency to gossip. After all, *nothing* is too big or too small for Him to care about. He is a real '90s kind of Guy. He knows what is pressuring teens today, and He is willing to help if you will let Him.

In a perfect world, everyone would treat one another as they themselves wish to be treated—with respect, affection, and courtesy. What's more, boys and girls could actually be friends without letting jealousy, possessiveness, sex, or any other complication get in the way.

But, as much as we'd like that (and should strive for it anyway), this is *real life* and it's not perfect. That's what *Dear Judy . . . Did You Ever Like a Boy (Who Didn't Like You?)* is about—handling real-life problems that real teens encounter.

You've asked me these questions. Together we'll try to figure out the answers. So here goes. . . .

PART I

Friendships

● ● ● ● ● ● ● ● ●

*Some friends may ruin you. But a real friend will be
more loyal than a brother.*

Proverbs 18:24

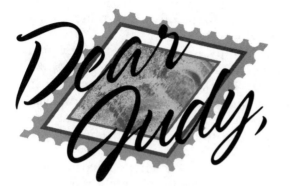

"When We Moved I Thought I'd Die..."

● ● ● ● ● ● ● ● ●

I moved to a new state last month. It was a really hard move. I had to leave a lot of close friends. I cry almost every night because I miss everyone so much. I don't have any friends here and I've been depressed lately. I can put myself in Lexi's place and understand how she feels. After reading the book New Girl In Town, *I realized that if I give this place a chance it might not turn out to be so bad after all. It can never replace my old home, but I can still keep in touch with my old friends and make new ones here.*

—Sonya

Exactly!

Attitude is everything when you are in a situation that's out of your control.

As the old saying goes, "When life gives you lemons, make lemonade." Turn the sour and bitter parts of your life into something sweet. It won't always be simple or easy, but it is *possible*.

Although it feels overwhelming right now, you have a

major opportunity to take charge of your own life. *Choose not to let this get you down.*

I like to be around happy, upbeat people, don't you? I seek them out and avoid crabby, whiny ones. *So be someone others want to be around!* Think of all the things you *like* in a person (friendliness, enthusiasm, courtesy, kindness, willingness to be a good sport . . .) and strive for those qualities in yourself. It will be great practice for the remainder of your life.

And what if it doesn't work out? That's a learning experience too. Persist. Get involved—join a church group or a sports team, see what school organizations interest you. . . .

Be someone others want to be around! Think of all the things you like in a person and strive for those qualities in yourself.

But watch out. Being *too* eager scares people off too. *Be cool and *stay* cool*—even if that's not what you feel inside. A person who is too panicked and too eager sends off signs of desperation. You might as well yell into a crowded room, "Be my friend, *please!*"

You don't have to be desperate. Do you know why? Because you're too good for that! You are a unique, one-of-a-kind, nobody-else-quite-like-you person. Don't sell yourself short. You *may* have to spend some time alone. That's okay. It's far better than rushing to make friends and doing things that you may regret later.

I'm moving to a new town. I'm nervous because I'm usually a victim of cliques. I'm not ugly, but I'm always the new girl, unwanted and unneeded.

—Marla

Let's rewrite that last sentence. How does this sound? "I'm the new girl, *intriguing and exciting.*" That could be a true statement too, you know. Sometimes the new girl is the most interesting girl in school because she comes from a different place, has new experiences to share, and is a change from the same old familiar faces at school. Just because you're new doesn't mean you're unwanted and unneeded. Don't move into town expecting the worst—or you may find it!

What interests you? Music? Church activities? Sports? Get involved! Don't sit around waiting for someone to take you under their wing. Get out and meet people halfway. Besides, it's more fun to be friends with an active, upbeat person than one who looks like their pet hamster just died.

Sometimes being the new girl isn't so bad. After all, you've got new, exciting experiences to share!

One more suggestion—*be patient.* Friendships don't happen overnight. They take time to take root and grow. You have to remember that your future best friend may be exactly like you are right now—and holding back to see what *you* will do. So reach out!

Like Lexi in your first Cedar River Daydreams book, New Girl In Town, *I had to move to a new town. The girls were mean—especially the one in power. As soon as I set foot in the classroom, they all giggled and gave me funny looks. When I came home from school I'd cry and think how much I hated it here.*

I made friends with a bunch of older girls, but they went boy-crazy and did a lot of things they shouldn't have done. I was with them all the way. I feel so stupid for being pulled into that horrid mess. When my mom found out what we'd been up to, she wouldn't allow me to see them anymore. I miss all my friends back home and I cry a lot.

—May

Your problem isn't surprising or unusual. This happens to many girls who move. Still, you're at the new school to stay. Now you must focus on what you can do to improve your situation.

There must be another group (or perhaps just one other girl) who is more like you. No doubt that "girl in power" (Who gave her the "power" anyway?) has trounced on others' feelings before you came along. Perhaps some-one else is sick of revolving in this girl's orbit and would like to have a new friend too. It's up to you to find her.

Don't just be a follower. You're a unique, wonderful individual—so be confident in your own abilities.

Why is it that girls seem to give so much "power" to one or two leaders in a group? I've never quite understood how this happens, but through a combination of intimidation, boldness, and manipulation, one or two people in a class will often "rise to the top" as leaders and power brokers and manage to cause all sorts of trouble and heartache for others.

The girl who is manipulative and controlling is able to be that way because others allow her to do so. Someone can't lead if there are no followers. Teenagers should have more confidence in themselves and the unique, wonderful individuals that they are. Then they wouldn't be so willing to follow in the tracks of someone they think of as popular.

And about your statement "I cry a lot," crying is not always bad. After all, a little crying relieves tension. But, if you do it too long, too hard, and too often you need to quit. Get busy. Baby-sit. Take a class at the YWCA. See if there is a nursing home or library that would appreciate your volunteer services. Tough times pass; really they do.

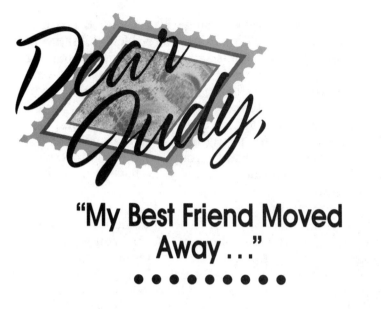

TWO

"My Best Friend Moved Away..."

●●●●●●●●●

My best and dearest friend in the world has moved away. It was awful. I miss her SO much. It still hurts at times, I mean REALLY hurts. There will never be another friend like her. We had so much in common and now she's gone. There's an awful hurt deep inside of me longing for the good times we had. I'll remember and treasure them forever, but it won't be the same.

—Dinah

I'm sorry to hear your friend has moved away and left you so lonely. That hurts. It takes a long time to get over the loneliness—and sometimes the memories come back when you least expect it.

Frankly, it might take quite a while before you find new people to fill the void left when your friend moved. But you've already begun to heal. You've accepted the move and realized that changes in your life will occur. ("I'll remember the good times and treasure them forever, but it won't be the same.")

I can't even tell you how many times friends of mine

have moved away. It *does* change everything. It can certainly ruin your social life until you are able to fill the void in your life with new friends and activities. It is like starting over—only your friend gets to "start over" in a brand-new place, and you are stuck in the familiar and, therefore, not-nearly-as-exciting old one!

It takes special effort to make new friends in a place where you've lived for a long time. The reason? Most everyone already has their "group." When your friend moved, it left you all alone and now you have to break into a new crowd.

How do you do this?

First of all, force yourself to do something new, something you haven't tried before. Maybe you've always thought of going out for golf, track, or tennis, but just have never gotten around to it. Sign up! Try it. You'll meet people there that you might not have met otherwise.

Call someone you've always liked but have never known very well. Ask them if they'd like to do something—shop, go for a walk, swim, whatever. You've probably been so engrossed with your other friend that you didn't notice the congenial overtures others have made toward you. Now is the time to tune yourself in to other people's thoughts and feelings.

Have a slumber party for the girls who are left behind. (Once, when several of my friends moved out of town within a short period of time and I was attending a lot of "Going Away" parties, I threatened to have a "Staying Here" party for those of us who were left!)

Even long-distance friendships can last a lifetime.

Don't lose touch with your friend even though she is gone. You can always exchange letters or postcards. Occasionally, I give my girls permission to call their friends long distance. I don't mind as long as they ask first and don't talk too long or too often. I know how important it is to hear a warm, familiar voice on the other end of the telephone line.

Perhaps you can visit her someday. Realistically, however, if you *do* visit, don't be disappointed if you can't pick up at exactly the same spot in your lives as when you last saw each other. You may grow apart. Be prepared for that. On the other hand, you may have a friendship that will survive the distance and span a lifetime. Cherish the memories—and make new, even more wonderful ones.

THREE

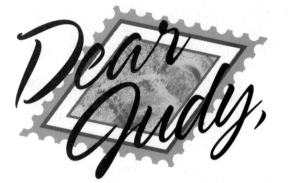

"I'm Starting a New School and I'm Scared..."

●●●●●●●●●

We moved from the East Coast to the West just a few days ago . . . I'm scared about starting school here. I was home-schooled in my old home.

—Linda

Our family is going to move soon. I'm a little shy so I'm worried about what it will be like to make all new friends.

—Deana, age 12

I'm eleven years old and just moved to a new city. I'm going to start middle school and I'm a little scared. I don't know anyone.

I used to be really popular at my old school, but I don't know how to make friends here. I'm really shy most of the time. At my old school I always had friends and never had a problem with that. It's going to be different now. I just know it.

My mom says I'll have no problem because everyone my age is just starting middle school. It's not that easy. Everyone else has friends from elementary school. I don't know what to do. Alexis

Leighton and I have a lot in common. I used to have friends like the Hi-Fives. Then I moved.

—Joyce, age 11

It *is* scary! And hard. And sometimes just awful. Frankly, *I* still get nervous in a new group. I don't like walking into a room where I don't know a single person. In situations like that, I feel as if everything I say is dumb and insignificant.

But even though I *feel* this way, having those feelings doesn't make it a fact. I probably don't sound as stupid as I think I do (at least I hope not!). What's more, there is probably someone, somewhere in the group, who is actually interested in meeting me. It will be that way for you too.

Relax! Don't look for trouble. New situations can be a lot of fun!

After all, you said yourself that you were "really popular" at your old school. Why shouldn't you eventually be popular at your new school, too?

What did people like about you? Were you friendly? Funny? Generous? Kind? It worked once without your having to try too hard. It should work again.

You are so sure that something awful is going to happen that it probably will. Reread your words: *"It's going to be different now. I just know it."* Your negative mind-set might make it so by changing the really terrific person you actually are. I know this is going to be difficult, but *relax*! Go into this new situation optimistically.

I like to be around people who smile easily and often, who are kind and considerate, who are truly interested in me. I'm less enthusiastic about people who are self-involved or too worried about making an impression to relax and be themselves. Aren't you? Remember that the first day of school and things will work out.

I am exactly like Lexi. I am the new girl at school. It is hard at first, but when you're at the bottom there is nowhere to go but up.

—Wendy

I like your attitude! It's both *realistic* and *optimistic*. You see the facts as they really are (although being the new girl at school isn't the total bottom!), but you also look for the best yet to come. You'll do fine in your new school.

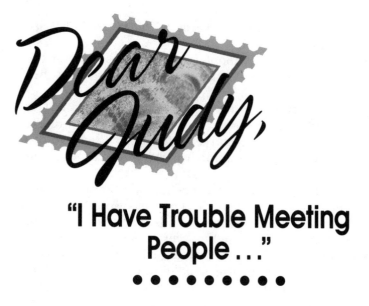

FOUR

"I Have Trouble Meeting People..."

● ● ● ● ● ● ● ● ●

I am twelve years old. I have trouble when I meet new people. I don't know how to get to know them. Do you have any ideas? Also, I would like an interesting idea on how to get along with my friends.

—Libby, age 12

Friendships are forged when people work or play together. What's more, it's easier to get to know people in small groups rather than in large ones.

Speak to people! That sounds so simple that it's almost silly, but it's good advice. Have you ever wished to visit with someone you found interesting but didn't say a word for fear of being rejected or embarrassed? I know I have! But you'll never get to know someone if you don't talk to them. *Ask a question* to break the ice and see where it leads.

If you can't think of a question to ask, give the person a compliment. Everyone likes to hear, "I love your haircut," or "Where did you get that great sweater?" (or headband, or lipstick, or black eye—you get the idea). Your compliment must be genuine, however. Others can easily see through false flattery.

People love to talk about themselves. Give them the opportunity! Show enthusiasm and interest in what they are saying.

Reach out! Invite someone (or several someones) to watch TV, study, make cookies, or ride horseback. Engage your mom's help if necessary. Perhaps she'll help you to organize a pizza party, a slumber party, or a shopping trip to the mall.

One of the best "ice breakers" at our house was our little hand-held movie camera. The girls would set it up and film themselves and their friends singing, even doing skits and plays. By the time they were done planning what they would film, finding the needed costumes and music, writing the script, doing the actual filming, and rewinding the tape to watch the results, everyone was relaxed and happy. Maybe you don't own a video camera, but there are other equally creative ways to have fun.

The key to making—and keeping—friends is *Be Friendly*!

Keeping friends takes work too. It means being thoughtful when you don't feel like it, courteous and patient when you want to bop someone on the head, and kind when you'd really like to lash out and be cruel.

Friends your age (12) often fight among themselves. Don't be drawn into the problem. It's far better to be known as the neutral one, the one who refuses to take sides and hurt someone's feelings. Who needs to fight anyway? It's far more hassle than it's worth!

The best way to have friends is to *be* a friend. Treat people the way you want to be treated. It's hard not to like a person who seems genuinely interested in you. Ask questions. Smile. Make others feel special.

I have moved many times in my life. It's hard to make new friends. Some of the people I thought were my friends were not.

—Millie

That happens to adults, too. It really hurts when a friend disappoints you. That's why it's smart not to depend on just one person for all your friendship needs. Enjoy what is good about each of your friends, but don't expect them to be perfect. Then, when something happens and you are disappointed by what someone said or did, you will be able to cope with it more easily. It isn't nearly so devastating when there are others to turn to for comfort and company.

Have you ever heard the saying "Don't put all your eggs into one basket"? That means, don't depend on just one person to fulfill all your hopes and dreams. Spread your friendship around. That way, if your friend disappoints you (drops your basket), you (and your eggs) won't be totally crushed!

If Friend A is funny and friendly but has a terrible habit of borrowing things and not returning them, enjoy laughing with her but make it a policy never to lend her your things. If Friend B is the sweetest person in the world but so dizzy she drives you nuts, remember that your reward for putting up with a little dizziness is her warmth and kindness. If Friend C is exuberant and a kick to spend time with but can't keep a secret for anything, enjoy your time with her but *never* tell her anything you don't want the entire world to know. Know your friends' weaknesses and strengths. Then when something happens and you are disappointed by what someone said or did, you will be able to cope with it more easily. It isn't nearly so devastating when there are others to turn to for comfort and company.

My mother always told me that if I had one or two really good friends in my life I'd be lucky. She meant the kind of friend who understands you even when you aren't talking; the kind who is on your side through thick and thin; the kind you can talk to every day for the rest of your life and never get bored.

I thought that having only two of those friends sounded like too few. It worried me. I always met people with this thought floating in the back of my mind; "Are *you* going to be the one? Are you going to be a real friend?"

What my mother *really* meant was that although I would have lots of acquaintances and friendships with people I valued, I'd only find a few with that very special bond that would make us inseparable even when we were miles apart.

I didn't find my best friends until I was grown up. The first I met when I was nineteen years old. Talk about a bond! What wonderful talks we had! What laughter! What trust! By the way, I married my first best friend.

Enjoy what is good about each of your friends, but don't expect them to be perfect.

I found my next best friends after I started writing. For the first time in my life, I met people who were as passionately interested in the written word as I was. We had things in common that others didn't know or care about. We had similar values, beliefs, and attitudes. We "clicked."

I tell you this so that you might understand that there is no need to panic if you aren't the most popular person in school. It's okay. If, in your lifetime, you find only a few people with whom you really "connect" that's okay. Quality, not quantity, is important where friendship is concerned.

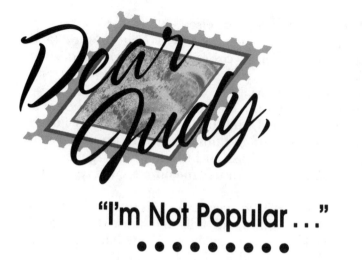

FIVE

"I'm Not Popular..."

● ● ● ● ● ● ● ● ●

Lexi has a popular boy as a friend, but Lexi just isn't that popular. It doesn't really work that way at my school. All the popular guys only like popular girls. I like a boy who is popular. He'll smile at me, wave to me, and talk to me when he's not with his friends.

—Shari

Some of my friends only like me because of my stuff and clothes.

—Faith

Ironic, isn't it, that in the Cedar River Daydreams series Minda Hannaford and her friends (who no one *really* likes very well) are considered popular. Lexi (who people like a great deal) isn't part of the "in" or "popular" crowd. I think it is that way for many teenagers today. Popularity sometimes means something other than being well liked by large numbers of people. Instead, it may mean being manipulative and intimidating enough to convince people that "you had better like me—or else!"

Popularity is often achieved by having outward (and sometimes superficial) successes such as a pretty face, good hair, lots of money, a nice car, a cute boyfriend, an outstanding talent that everyone admires . . .

True popularity—the kind that remains after the car is gone, the head is bald, and the face is wrinkled—is gained by having the inward (and not superficial) traits that mature people value. Those include kindness, generosity, thoughtfulness, respect for self and others, good spirit, and honesty.

In Cedar River Daydreams, Minda is superficially popular. Lexi, on the other hand, is liked because she is a good friend. Teenagers can often be shallow about who and what they like. So can adults. But I'd still rather have people like me because of my personality and good humor than because of the number of outfits in my closet!

I intentionally wrote the Cedar River Daydreams books with Todd and Lexi as a couple. I created Todd to be mature enough to recognize a girl's real best qualities (her mind, her values, her personality).

Do you really think much of a boy who will only speak to you when more popular people aren't around? Sounds like he still has some growing up to do. I wouldn't bother with him. You are special. You have value. God created only *one* of you. You deserve to be treated with respect and courtesy.

You are no less of a person because you don't have a boyfriend. It is far more pleasant to spend time with your friends than with a boy who puts you down or treats you as second rate.

I'm not that ugly but, of course, I'm not pretty either.

—Carmen, age 10

My dad is a pastor. The kids at school don't really accept me because I don't wear the clothes like they wear and I have an overbite. It's weird having friends over because when I introduce them to my dad they get embarrassed.

—Maggie, age 12

I'm sure that pastors' kids have special problems unique to them. After all, by being a P.K., you come with a built-in set of expectations. People might assume that because of who your father or mother is you are more religious or even that you consider yourself better than "regular" kids. Sometimes these high expectations cause P.K. s to rebel just to show how normal they really are.

Understand that your dad might be something of a mystery to your friends. Perhaps they haven't had the opportunity to attend church as often as you have. Though this attitude is your friends' problem, it becomes yours.

Your dad is the best person to help you with this situation.

After all, his job is to work with people. He should know better than anyone how to make others feel comfortable. Ask him for advice. Together, create a plan to put your friends at ease.

What might that plan be? That's up to you, but here are some suggestions:

1. Have him do something "dad-like" with your friends (shoot hoops, play softball); have a barbecue and ask your dad to do the cooking; work on a group science project together . . .
2. Let your friends see your dad in "regular" clothes (like blue jeans and an old sweatshirt), not "work" clothes (like a clerical collar and suit).

Even pastors were teenagers once—and they are human. If your friends realize that, they may be more comfortable around your dad.

Now, about those clothes you mentioned:

I don't know what you wear, but I really do believe that if you are beautiful on the inside that will outshine whatever you wear on the outside. Still, it is uncomfortable to be totally out of step with your peers.

You do have to go along with what your parents wish as far as clothing is concerned, but perhaps you can ask to have more input into your wardrobe. (Only you will know if this suggestion is appropriate or not.) When it is time to get something new, shop with your mom and look for things in which you will feel more comfortable. Be patient—it takes a while to revamp a wardrobe.

Remember, the clothes you wear are just the package—the gift is inside!

Being scrupulously clean and neat are very important, of course. Do the best you can with what you have and then *relax* and forget about your clothing. Personality means much more than clothing anyway.

The overbite is another story. That's really a dental problem that must be solved between your family and your dentist.

In the meantime, remember that you'll be *more* conspicuous if you are always trying to keep your mouth closed or cover it with your hand. Smile. Laugh. That's what people will remember most about you.

Physical appearance is only a small part of what makes people view you as attractive.

Think of your favorite people in the whole world, the ones with whom you like best to spend time.

Are they all beautiful?

Are they all perfect?

Are they all without a flaw of any kind?

Of course not!

But you're crazy about them anyway, right?

See what I mean?

You are liked or disliked for many reasons—not only on the basis of your physical appearance. While you may not be able to change your appearance (other than to make sure you are always perfectly clean and well-groomed), you can change other things that might prevent you from making new friends. In the friendship business, personality counts. Work on having a nice one.

It seems that Lexi has an easy time making friends. She's the exact opposite of me.

—Denise

I like sports. Actually, what I like best is being on the team. I am short and not a very good player so most people don't want to play with me.

—Jeanette

I would like it if you would answer my letter when you get the time. I'm not popular, but if I had a letter with your signature on it, I would be. If you could help me by writing to me, I will be more than your friend, I will be other people's friend, too.

—Tammy, age 13

I am not the most popular girl in my school. In fact, I am one of the least *popular. I can't do anything with my hair. My face is continually breaking out. Even though I go to a Christian school, when I try to act like a Christian I am kicked out of everything. I've never had a real boyfriend and I'm always picked last for teams in phy. ed. I'm really lonely and there's no one to sympathize with me or help me. I've prayed about it and that helps. Your books encourage me too, and I haven't gotten depressed or lonely enough to do anything drastic.*

—Lisa, age 14

Every single person on the face of the earth has felt lonely or misunderstood at one time or another. Sometimes people disappoint you or don't seem to understand what is going on in your mind.

Unfortunately, you sound *really* down about the situation you are in and I think it is important that you *take action* immediately. First of all, *find someone to talk to!* Where are your mom and dad? Do you have an older sister, an aunt, a neighbor in whom you could confide? Just having someone listen to you will probably make you feel better. (If you ever feel like doing yourself harm, *run*, don't walk, to the nearest help you can find—your parents, your pastor, your teacher or guidance counselor. Tell them exactly how you've been feeling. Ask them to help you. Don't try to hide your feelings.)

True popularity—the kind that remains after the car is gone, the head is bald, and the face is wrinkled—is gained by having the inward traits that people value.

Your physical problems are more easily changed. Perhaps you should ask someone to take you to get a really good haircut—the kind that looks great as long as it's kept washed and combed. Also, a dermatologist or even your family physician can help you get that skin problem under control. Managing these physical things should make you feel more in control mentally.

Next, *take a look at your attitude.* You sound gloomy and "poor me" right now. Is that attitude helping you to make friends or driving potential friends away? We all like to be around cheerful, upbeat people. Even if you don't feel like it, try to smile and be pleasant. It will be difficult, I know, but sometimes when I'm in a lousy mood, if I have to *act* happy for others, I actually begin to *feel* happier inside. Crazy, but it sometimes works.

Fortunately for us, we do have a friend who *always* understands us! When things go wrong, you can always share your thoughts, your ideas, your frustrations with Jesus. He'll be there to listen and to help you over the rough spots in your life. He's your friend forever. Hebrews 13:5 promises, "I will never leave you or forsake you." And God never lies!

New Girl In Town *taught me a good lesson. When you're under peer pressure you sometimes do stupid and sick things, but you don't have to do them.*

—Vickie, age 11

Everyone wants to be popular at school and everyone wants to be nice. People usually end up being only one or the other, but Lexi is both.

—Brittany

It might be hard, but I do think you can be both. Perhaps you won't be the "absolutely most popular girl in town," but you can be well liked. I like to be around people who make me feel good about being me. I like people who are easy to talk to, who listen to what I say with interest, who make me feel like I'm special. I also like people who are real and honest, who don't pretend to be something or someone they're not. I like to know that when a person leaves me, she doesn't go to someone else to talk about me behind my back. I like a person who cares about me. Who wouldn't?

And how do you get to *be* that kind of person? By thinking less about yourself (Is my hair all right? Does he think I'm cute?) and thinking more about *others* (making sure they are comfortable, included in the conversation, whatever). Build up the people around you. Be secure and willing to share the glory or attention of the moment.

Popularity that depends on cruelty, exclusion, or power-plays won't last forever. Popularity based on a genuinely kind and caring attitude will.

I have a friend who wants to be popular, but the popular girls are like the Hi-Fives. They talk about you behind your back. Now they are trying to get me to turn against her but I think she's nice. I want to know what to do.

—Corina, age 11

You like her. She's your friend. You obviously don't want to lose her as a friend or you would never have written to me! Therefore, don't be forced into turning against her by a group of girls who don't sound as though they are even very nice!

Think of it this way—what if *you* were the girl they were

talking about? How would you want your friend to behave toward you? You'd want her to be loyal, wouldn't you? You'd be terribly hurt if she turned against you. Treat her in the way you would like to be treated.

Why do you want to be friends with those girls anyway? What if you actually do what they've asked? Do you have any promise that you won't be their *next* target?

I really liked the fact that Lexi stood up to the Hi-Fives and refused to shoplift. That must have been hard when she wanted to have friends. Still, she didn't let them talk her into it. I probably would have let them push me around and done things for them so I could be with the popular group. Most of my friends would probably do the same thing. New Girl in Town *showed me that I need to learn to stand up to people. I have learned some great lessons through your books. Thanks a lot.*

—Lynn, age 12

I think everyone at one time or another has been pushed into doing something they really didn't approve of because they wanted to be liked or accepted by a group or another person. We have a strong need to be liked and accepted. It's easy to think that if we do or say everything others want us to, we will become part of the group. In reality, it doesn't always work that way.

Sometimes, people will test you. They will use you as a "go-fer." "Go-fer a can of pop and bring back some chips while you're at it." You are really more of a servant than a friend. Are you willing to do that just to be a part of the "popular" group?

Popularity that depends on cruelty, exclusion, or power-plays won't last forever. Popularity based on a kind and caring attitude will.

What's more, sometimes you'll be asked to do things that you don't approve of (It happened to Lexi in *New Girl in Town*). It's one thing to be a doormat for kids who want you to run errands for them. It's another to smoke, swear, steal, tease, ridicule others, or whatever else your "friends" want you to do in order to be accepted by their group.

You have some decisions to make. When you are asked to do something that you really don't want to do, ask yourself this question: "How will I feel later? Will I feel guilty? cheap? stupid? disappointed in myself?" If your answer is yes to any of these questions, *don't do it!* It's not worth sacrificing your self-esteem to be popular.

How do you say no? It can be hard, especially when you are the only one refusing to go along with the crowd. Often the best way to diffuse an uncomfortable situation is with a light touch.

Let's say, for example, that everyone in your group is smoking but you. You could

1. give them all a big lecture about the dangers of tobacco and secondhand smoke and make everyone think you're a real prude.
2. say, "No thanks. My dad can smell smoke a mile away. He won't let me hang around with you guys if he thinks we're smoking. I'll pass. I'd rather not be grounded for life."
3. say pleasantly, "Not now. I'm not into that. Are there any chips left?"

Most parents are willing to be the "bad guys" for their children. If you don't want to do something, it's effective to say that you'll be in trouble at home if you take part in the questionable behavior (and it's true, right? You *will* be in trouble at home). What's more, parents understand that sometimes it's easier for a teenager to say, "My parents won't let me," than it is to say, "I won't let myself." When you are strong enough, you will be able to face any situation and say, "I don't approve and I won't participate." If you find yourself in circumstances in which it is hard to say no, let Mom or Dad (or the threat of their presence) say no for you.

Also remember that if you don't make a big deal of

saying no, maybe no one else will either. If you give a big lecture and then run from the room, you're going to have a different response than if you calmly say no and then ask someone to pass the chips! Try to stay cool and calm. It helps. (Of course, if the group is doing *a lot* of things you don't approve of, you shouldn't be there anyway. Get away as gracefully as possible.)

Hard as it may be to believe, others *respect* people who are individuals and who stand up for their beliefs. You don't have to follow the crowd. You are great just the way you are. Some of my favorite people are true *individuals*— they don't care what anyone else thinks. I admire their bravery, their self-confidence, and their uniqueness.

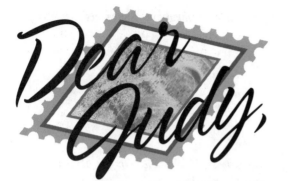

SIX

"All I Want Is One Good Friend—Just One..."

● ● ● ● ● ● ● ● ●

I've prayed all year to find a good friend—boy or girl. All I've found are problems, trouble, and heartache. All I want is one good friend, just one!

I know I don't know you, but after I read your book I felt like I could tell you this. It felt good to tell my problems to someone I wasn't related to...

P.S. Sorry my letter is sloppy, but I was kinda nervous telling you this!!!

—Linnea, age 14½

The reason I'm writing to you and telling you everything is that I have no friends and haven't had since I moved. I am so lonesome that I feel like Lexi did in New Girl in Town. *It feels great to write you! Knowing I've got a new friend makes me happy!*

—Mari, age 13

Is there a real Lexi, Todd, Harry, Peggy and the rest of the gang? I would love to meet a girl like Lexi. I scarcely have any friends in school, only two.

—Judith

My mom teaches me at home. I don't have any friends except those in church and in gymnastics.

—Ardyth, age 13

The only thing I want is friends who wait for me after school and call me a lot—not just every other week.

—Denni

Much of my mail is from girls who desperately want a friend. They have a great need to belong. It may not help much to know this, but, for those of you who are lonely, you aren't the only person in the world with this problem!

Give people both time and room to get to know you. Let them see for themselves that you can be compassionate, affirming, relaxing, and fun to be around.

I believe that the *majority* of teenagers feel alone and lonely at least part of the time. Young people are notorious for changing friends and for "trying on" new relationships for a while and then discarding them. It's all part of the self-discovery process through which teenagers go. (I didn't say this was *easy*, but I do believe it's *normal!*)

You are traveling through a very unstable, unpredictable time in life. Though a friend would be a great help, you might not find that *BFF* (Best Friend Forever) you've been looking for.

Then what?

Talk to your mom. Tell her you're lonely. Ask her to help you think of new ways to meet people. Church or gymnastics are good. So are Girl Scouts, 4-H, a bowling league, sports, or an activity at the YWCA. Invite people over to study or do a school project. You will have to decide what is appropriate for you.

REACH OUT! Find others in your school who are lonely too. Perhaps there is a new girl in school or someone who appears to be alone a great deal. Seek these people out. Be friendly and be creative.

Warning: Don't behave as though you are desperate to have a friend. Others will find that alarming and you might scare them away. You will make them wonder why you are so terribly eager to make a friend. They may even begin to wonder what's 'wrong' with you.

Give people both time and room to get to know you. Let them see for themselves that you can be fun and funny, compassionate and affirming, enjoyable and relaxing to be around.

Lexi is so down-to-earth and sensible about everything. I love the fact that she believes in God and mentions Him often, because I do too! I wish she lived in my neighborhood! I would love to have someone to go to with my problems who I was sure would help me.

I also like her friends. I wish I had friends like that. All the kids here don't really care about each other like Lexi and her friends do.

—Quinn

We could all take some lessons from Lexi about being a friend. She *is* "down-to-earth and sensible." She's also kind, caring, compassionate, a good sport, tolerant, patient, pleasant, and loving. She has both talents and flaws.

Perhaps the most important thing to do to gain friends is to learn how to *be* a friend. Think of the qualities you've noticed in yourself, and then in the people around you. Are they crabby? cheerful? selfish? shallow? sullen? smiley? good listeners? nonstop talkers? childish? insecure? optimistic? pessimistic? friendly? petty? bossy? eager to please? pouty? negative? upbeat? gossipy? dishonest? good-hearted? sensitive? calm? excitable?

Add whatever characteristics you've observed in others.

Now pick out the traits you like best. Circle them with a pencil. Study them. This is a picture of your idea of a good friend.

Here comes the hard part—make an effort to incorporate those qualities into your own life and to weed out the characteristics you don't like. If you did this, you would be a great friend to have!

There's a verse in the Bible that says it well. "A person should live so that he pleases the Lord. If he does, even his enemies will make peace with him" (Proverbs 16:7).

Of course, even the most cheerful person in the world has down days. It's *how* you handle your crabby mood that will make the difference. On more than one occasion when I've been stressed to my limit and in no mood to be pleasant, I've told my family, "This is a warning. I'm cranky today. It's not your fault, but I'd recommend not doing anything to upset me. Tread softly!"

I'd never intentionally snap at someone in my family, but if they've had fair warning they are less likely to take it personally. Besides, I might even find a sympathetic ear, someone who says, "What's bugging you, Mom?" And if they listen nicely, I might be cajoled out of my crabby mood.

Here's another tip straight from the Bible about friendship: "A friend loves you all the time. A brother is always there to help you" (Proverbs 17:17). That's what friendship is all about!

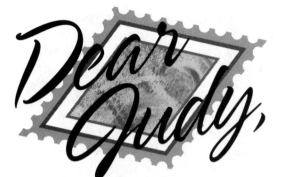

SEVEN

With Friends, Three's Usually a Crowd

●●●●●●●●●

I used to have a best friend back in fourth grade. Now that we're in fifth, we don't have a lot in common and keep getting into fights. We tried to stay together, but it didn't work out, so we broke up. Then Nadine started playing with Denise (my other very good friend). Now they won't pay any attention to me. Nadine and Denise both say they're still my friends, but they never talk to me, and ignore me. I discussed this with my parents. They said that everything would be fine and that I should try to make new friends, but it never works out.

I tried to make new friends, but they don't like me. I get really lonely at school and wonder why this had to happen to me. I'm having a hard time right now. Could you give me some advice on what I should do? I'm telling you this because most of the books you write have the problems that children face. You seem to understand these problems better than all the other people I know because I've already talked to them and all they tell me is to be patient. But I don't think I can stand this much longer.

—Erin, age 10

The way I see it, you have at least two choices.

First, you could confront Nadine and Denise and tell them how you feel and try to work it out. Perhaps they don't know how hurt you feel and don't realize how their behavior is affecting you. This is a difficult choice to make, but if you want to maintain the friendship it might help.

Secondly, you could decide to accept the situation. Nadine and Denise will be closer to each other than they are to you. Ouch! That hurts! But, if that's what happens, try to be tolerant. If you lash out at them, that will certainly drive them away and lessen the possibility that they'll begin including you again. Perhaps you and your friends have outgrown each other. Find other ways to be busy and involved.

When things get tough, talk to Jesus. You'll be surprised at how good it feels to voice your problems to Him.

You said, "I *tried* to make friends, but they don't like me." Friends can't be made overnight. Friendship is a slow, gradual process. People often become friends when they have the same interests or work together on projects. True friendships take time to develop. I know that seems hard, especially when you need a friend so much, but don't panic. And don't be negative. That's a real turn-off for most people.

I wish I had a simple, easy answer for you, but I don't. Life can be very difficult and complicated. But don't worry. There *is* a friend out there for you. You just haven't met her yet. Remember, we've always got a heavenly Friend to talk to, and He's a great listener.

I have a problem. I have two good friends, but they don't get along very well sometimes! When I'm friends with one of them the other one gets mad. She'll get lots of my other friends on her side and gang up on me! Do you know what I could do? I hope you have some answers for me!

—Gigi

I have two wonderful best friends, but they're jealous of each other. When I talk to one the other gets mad! What should I do?

—Vicki, age 10

Three playmates or friends never seem to work out as well as two. Even when my children were tiny, I preferred that they have an even-numbered group of playmates. That way, everybody would have "somebody" and no one would be left out. Kids aren't very sophisticated about including everyone in their play (even some adults are very territorial and don't like to "share" their friends).

Everyone, at some time or another, has felt the pain of that three-is-a-crowd experience . . . knowing that it is common might make you a little more patient.

You may end up being the peacemaker between your friends. Can you make them both understand that you like them equally well? That true friendship doesn't involve ganging up on someone to punish them? Otherwise, this problem may continue until you lose one or both of your friends—or everyone becomes mature enough to handle a three-way friendship.

When nothing else helps, sometimes the thing to do is just wait out your friend's anger. Something else will crop up to divert her attention. It's hard to stay mad forever. Hang in there!

A new girl, I'll call her Minda after the girl in your books, stole my best friend. She rode the same bus I did. When she quit riding the bus she said that it was because I had lice (and I didn't). That was a lie and it became a rumor. My best friend (I'll call her Katie) wouldn't hang around me anymore. She didn't even talk to me. Minda told lies about me and Katie believed her. The other girls would do stuff with me, but Katie doesn't do anything with me anymore. Katie is Minda's only real friend now. Minda even accused me of stealing her things, but I didn't. Since Minda is blaming me for all this, I have to change schools. What should I do?

—Faye

This is a tough one. The first thing I'd say is *stay away from Minda!* She sounds like bad news. Stealing is a serious accusation. Evidently, if you are changing schools, your parents have become involved in this situation. That's good. Sometimes kids try to handle too much on their own. That's what parents are for—to help you out when you need it!

Since the decision to change schools is already made, I think you should look at this as a new and wonderful opportunity to make new friends. It is a fresh start for you. Enjoy it. Make the most of it. Have fun. You deserve it.

My former best friend and I got into a fight. I was wondering if you could tell me who is more to blame. My best friend started hanging around with two other girls and leaving me behind. They're entering puberty and they think I and my other friends are immature because we aren't starting puberty yet. Amy and Sara are even talking about getting best-friend necklaces. AND I THOUGHT AMY AND I WERE BEST FRIENDS!

—Leslie

You sound terribly disappointed by your best friend. You are hurt and angry. That's perfectly natural. I doubt that starting puberty is a valid reason for breaking off a friendship—I have a hunch that there are other reasons for this disagreement as well. Can you talk calmly to your friend? Can you ask her what went wrong in your friendship?

You asked me to tell you "who was more to blame" in this instance. Placing blame doesn't really help. That will divide you even further. There is an interesting reference to friendship in the Bible that says, "Whoever forgives someone's sin makes a friend. But the one who tells about the sin breaks up friendships" (Proverbs 17:9). That sounds like good advice to me.

Tina and I have been great friends since sixth grade. We'd go to each other's houses every day. Every weekend she'd sleep over at my house or I'd go to hers. We had tons of things in common and always agreed on things. Almost. Things were going great until we got into eighth grade. Tina got involved with another friend of mine. Now Tina wants all three of us to be best friends. I want only one best friend. They spend more time together than with me. They sit together in class now. Whenever I call Tina, she's already made plans with my other friend. This really hurts me. They don't ignore me, but I feel left out. We are all together but what I really want is to have my best friend back. Judy, what should I do? I am totally lost here.

—Stacey

Tina is obviously giving you the message that she needs and wants *more* than one best friend. You may have to make a choice—to share Tina or to try and monopolize all her time and lose her completely as a friend.

It's a good sign that the other girls are not ignoring you. That's an indication that they don't intend to leave you out and that they really do want to spend time with you. Try relaxing for a couple of weeks and not getting upset with Tina or your other friend. Just enjoy them and the things you do together. Maybe you will find that it works out after all.

We can't "own" people or require that they restrict their friendships to please us. That's asking too much of a person and could ruin an otherwise perfectly nice friendship.

Don't put Tina in a position in which she has to choose between you and your other friend. Someone will be badly hurt if you do that—and it could be you.

You've probably guessed by now that there are no easy

answers to questions about friendship. Every person is unique and has different needs and expectations to be fulfilled. Your desire is to have only *one* best friend. Tina wants *two*. You will have to work it out either in your own mind or with Tina. I hope that you will both try to understand the other's point of view. You've been friends too long to harm your friendship now.

There is nothing more disheartening or depressing than to lose a friend or to be lonely. Occasionally this happens. Hard as this may be to do, be patient. Sometimes the passage of time (which provides you with new opportunities to meet other people and find new interests) is the only thing that helps.

I have three close friends. I also have one major enemy, who is constantly saying bad things about me and putting me down. Sometimes I even feel that my friends aren't really my friends. I'll see one friend tell another something. Then they'll tell it to a third friend. I expect her to come and talk to me like she always used to but she doesn't. It makes me feel like I have no friends left. At lunch they hang all over each other and say, "Can I sit by you, please?" I end up sitting by myself at the other end of the table because there aren't any seats left by them. I see them laughing and having a good time without me.

Do you know any Bible verses that could help me or have any good advice? It's really awful feeling so alone.

—Sivanah

You aren't feeling very self-confident right now (maybe because of that "major enemy" who keeps putting you down). As a result, you're feeling distrustful and anxious about your other friends as well. When a person is unhappy, fears rejection, or is anxious about what others think about her, it shows. Try to be a little more confident around your friends. Be one of the first in line for lunch so that there *is* a seat for you at the table.

It sounds to me as though your friends aren't intentionally leaving you out. I suspect that since you are apprehensive about being excluded, you are behaving differently or holding back, waiting to be invited into a group that has already accepted you. This gets to be what's called a "vicious circle." The more left out you feel, the more withdrawn you'll act and the more left out you'll be. It's up to you to break the cycle.

The more left out you feel, the more withdrawn you'll act, and the more left out you'll be! Your attitude can stop the cycle.

If things get really bad, remember this verse: "The Lord defends those who suffer. He protects them in times of trouble. . . . He will not leave those who come to him" (Psalm 9:9–10). There is one Friend who never changes and never stops loving you. With Him, you can face any situation.

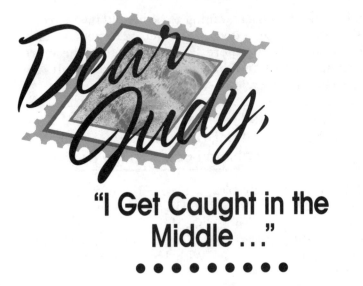

EIGHT

"I Get Caught in the Middle..."

●●●●●●●●●

I'm in the eighth grade. All my friends do is bicker and argue. It's hard being a Christian and having your friends act so awful and rebellious. I'm always stuck in the middle because I stay out of the stupid arguments. While I'm with one person, they really cut down my other friend. When I'm with that other person, I have to listen to it the other way around. They talk constantly about each other. Can you give me advice on helping my friends turn into Christians? My friends can't afford to go to a Christian camp and the churches here are hard to understand. I wish we had a teenager's church so everything would be on our level.

—Georgia, eighth grade

I'm glad that you don't get into the bickering and arguing with your friends! Have you ever *refused* to listen to the negative things they say about each other? Try saying, "I like both of you so much that I don't want to hear anything bad about either of you. Let's change the subject." Perhaps after you say that a few times your friends will get the idea that you aren't interested in hearing negative things and they'll stop running each other down.

In Matthew 5:14–16, the Bible says, "You are the light of the world. A city set on a hill cannot be hid. Nor do men light a lamp and put it under a bushel, but on a stand, and it gives light to all in the house. Let your light so shine before men, that they may see your good works and give glory to your Father who is in heaven."

The way to show your friends the Christian path is to be that "light." No matter what they might do or say, do not bicker or gossip. Show, by your actions, another way— Christ's way. That's what witnessing is all about—living your life in a special, appealing way that makes others "sit up and take notice." Make your friends wish that they, too, had your calm, your kindness, your compassion. You can then tell them where it comes from—God.

You can talk until you are blue in the face, but if your actions (impatience, rudeness, whatever) say something else, then you cannot be a good witness.

Perhaps there is an active youth group or youth ministry in which you can participate. There may be a Youth For Christ or Fellowship of Christian Athletes group in your area. They are both nondenominational. Check with your church or school to find out if there is such a group near you. Invite your friends. Showing what a Christian can do and be is far more effective than words alone!

I have a small problem. I've got three best friends—Polly, Jane, and Raye. Raye thinks she's my best friend but Polly is my real true B.F. Raye might get mad if I tell her that, but I know Jane won't. Raye is my boyfriend's cousin. If she gets mad at me, she might get him to break up with me. But Raye said she wouldn't do that because it might ruin our friendship. Raye is younger than me. She bosses me around a lot, but she thinks we're best friends. Sometimes it really gets to me. Maybe you could help me.

—Veronica

Dear Judy,

It seems to me that you are very lucky to have three good friends. I see no reason to upset any of your friends by telling them who is your favorite friend. After all, that might change from day to day! Let them know they are all special and precious to you, each in their own way.

I'm a big believer in enjoying what is best about a friend and being tolerant of his or her quirks and idiosyncracies (crazy little habits!). Nobody is perfect—maybe they have to put up with a few things they don't like about you either! If I had to be flawless in order to have friends, I'd be a very lonely person.

If Raye's bossiness really drives you wild, perhaps you will have to begin to stand up for yourself. If she tells you to do something that you don't want to do, politely refuse. Say that whatever it is she's asked of you makes you un-comfortable, unhappy, uneasy, whatever. Don't pick a fight. Just say no and change the subject. Eventually she'll get the idea.

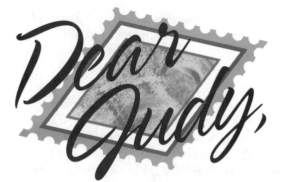

NINE

"How Do I Deal With Bullies?"

●●●●●●●●●

I have some problems at school. My friend is always bossing me around. She's kinda like Minda in your books.

—Alicia

There was a girl in my former hometown who made my life miserable. She decided she didn't like me so she turned everyone against me. I had no friends. Sounds like Minda Hannaford, doesn't it?

—Kaylee, age 13

There is a girl in my class who is almost like Minda. She and I have always been "natural enemies." We are always exchanging mean comments. After I read your book Trouble With a Capital T, *I tried to "turn the other cheek." We have really been getting along better.*

—Geri

I like Minda because she reminds me of a boy I know. He always picks on me. I also know a girl like Minda. I would like to punch this girl out.

—Viola

As you can tell from these excerpts from my mail, *everybody* has a "Minda" in his or her life. (Perhaps you have two or three Mindas with whom to contend!) Even the mean, bossy Minda-types have their own problems. There is bound to be someone, somewhere, able to handle every Minda and put her in her place!

Take comfort in the fact that we've all had this experience (yes, even me—lots of times!) and that it's something through which everyone manages to live.

Have you ever heard the phrase, "Like water off a duck's back"? Ducks, because they spend so much time in the water, have an oily substance in their feathers that makes water roll right off their bodies rather than seep through the feathers to create a very soggy and miserable duck. (Another one of God's outstanding creations!) So, when this nemesis of yours (that's the person who wants to be your undoing, to see your downfall—like Minda in the Cedar River Daydreams books) says something hurtful or cruel, let the words slide off you like water off a duck's back. Don't take the words to heart (don't get all soggy with misery). Your *attitude* will be your protection!

Once you aren't as much fun to harass (because of your new attitude), perhaps the troublemaker will leave you alone.

Minda and her friends (Tressa and Gina) are bullies. They like to be in control, to be the voice of authority. Why? I can't say in every case, but I'd guess that a lot of Minda-types are insecure. They aren't as perfectly confident as they'd like to have others believe. They only feel good when they feel popular and can make people jump to fulfill their wishes. They pick on people who might have just a little too much success, or people whom they see as weaker than themselves.

Minda-types usually stay away from confident, poised,

self-assured people who might put them in their place if they took their bullying too far.

Sometimes the Minda-types (and Tressa Williams from Cedar River Daydreams falls into this category) are just so sure that they are *right* and everyone else is *wrong* that they shove their opinions and attitudes down other people's throats. It's difficult to change anyone like that—only time and maturity will help (and sometimes even that doesn't do it!).

Never let someone pressure you into doing or saying something you don't want to do or say. Listen to your own conscience, your own inner voice.

It is important to stand up to the Minda-types. They'll never respect you otherwise. You can't make true friends by doing something that compromises your values.

On the other hand, don't listen to your desire to "punch her out" either. If a person becomes such a problem to you that you are considering violence, you'd better talk to your parents or a teacher and ask for their advice. You might need someone to "run interference" for you in order to settle the problem.

Some of the worst Minda-type people can grow up to be very nice people! Many people who were once viewed as bullies would be amazed and horrified to hear that fact once they reached adulthood! Every person finds his or her own way to get through the difficult childhood and teenage years. Even the Mindas struggle.

I hope that readers identify with Cedar River Daydreams, not in spite of Minda, but *because* of her! When she acts up and gives Lexi a hard time, the readers can nod and say "Yes! So-and-so did that very thing to me last week!" We all like to know that we aren't alone with our problems. It's comforting to realize that other people's lives aren't perfectly smooth either. Somehow it is easier to cope with a problem if you know others have it as well. We all have a Minda in our lives at one time or another—and we all live through it. Whew!

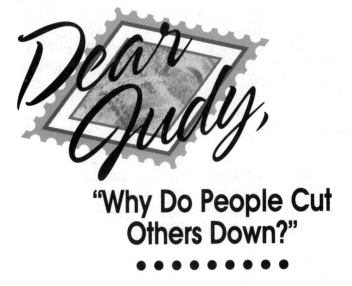

TEN

"Why Do People Cut Others Down?"

● ● ● ● ● ● ● ●

I don't understand why people are constantly cutting others down as a way to build themselves up when praising others would make them more popular.

—Corrinne

People who do this are functioning under the mistaken belief that if they cut others' accomplishments to shreds, they will look better as a result. Have you ever had a friend who simply couldn't say anything nice about anyone other than herself? Because she didn't feel good about herself, she felt threatened by anyone who did anything special or outstanding.

We have to remind ourselves that *just because someone else succeeds, it doesn't mean that we have failed.* Jealousy and envy are wicked things. They take away the pleasure we should have over our friends' successes.

It is very mature of you to realize that *praising* others is a far better tactic. It does indeed make you more popular than running others down. But it does something else as well. It makes you feel good inside.

I have a lot of wonderful, very successful writer friends. They receive many awards and accolades. When this happens, I have two choices: I could sneer and mutter under my breath, "Well, she's not *that* good. I really don't like her writing style. That award (or good review or high praise) must be just a fluke."

Instead of being jealous or envious of someone's achievement, I like to remind myself that if that good thing can happen to a friend of mine, it can happen to me!

Or, I could think, "Good for her! I'm so happy. It's time she was recognized for her good writing. Let's celebrate!"

I do the second. Frankly, it makes me feel wonderful to have such talented friends. I am truly proud of them. If I let jealousy and envy overtake me, I begin to feel small and withered inside. If I allow myself to be happy for another's successes, I feel generous, mature, and delighted that I'm fortunate enough to have a friend who can accomplish so much.

This is a choice we all must make. We can either cut others down and diminish ourselves in the process, or we can build others up and discover the joy that comes from celebrating with those we care about.

ELEVEN

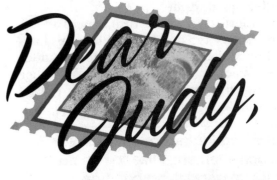

"People Make Fun of My Friend..."

● ● ● ● ● ● ● ● ●

What do you do if a different person is being made fun of?

1. *Should you ignore it if the kids making fun of her are rough?*
2. *Should you tell the kids to "back off" if they are rough?*
3. *Should you go tell an adult? Would that be dumb?*
4. *Should you ask your friends to help you?*
5. *Should you wait until they stop making fun and then tell them to leave her alone?*
6. *Should you break up the fight and run for it?*
7. *Should you just try to beat them up and knock them over?*
8. *Should you get your brother or sister to do the fighting?*
9. *Should you tell the principal privately?*
10. *Should you ask your mom and dad what to do?*

Would you please write me back very soon and tell me the good answer to the questions. I know it's difficult.

—Mandy, fourth grade

First, let me tell you a little story. Being a farm girl, I

was always particularly interested in animals. The chickens weren't my favorite creatures (not cuddly enough for my taste), but I did like the baby chicks. As they grew older, the chicks began to lose their fluffy yellow down. It was replaced by coarse white "adult" feathers. Occasionally the chickens would peck at one another with their beaks. These little beaks were sharp enough to break the skin and draw blood from the chicken they were picking on.

I learned that chickens *like* the sight of blood. Once a chicken is "down" or injured, the other chickens delight in picking at its wounds until they sometimes kill the poor "victim chicken." It is as though chickens, like human bullies, can pick out the weaker, not quite perfect individual in the bunch. And, just as human bullies often do, chickens will peck and peck and peck at the poor victim until they do hurtful, sometimes irreparable damage.

Yuk! you say? It is yukky. And gruesome. And it doesn't make you think very favorably of chickens either! Unfortunately, sometimes *people* (who have much bigger brains than chickens) do exactly the same type of thing. They pick on someone weaker and more helpless than themselves until they break the heart or spirit of another human being.

It is wise to have a plan of action in case you find yourself, or your friend, in trouble.

It's smart not to jump into a fight if you know the kids doing the teasing are rough and might actually do bodily harm to you or your friend. You'll have to be the judge of that situation. Only you will know if you are comfortable telling these bullies to "back off."

It's not dumb at all to tell an adult (the principal or a teacher or parent, for example) what is going on. In fact, it's probably one of your more intelligent choices. Bullies only like to bully when they won't get caught (that's because bullies are usually cowards). If you need protection, get it.

You are right to worry about your friend, and it is admirable that you wish to help him or her. There is no one good answer to this question. When you don't know what choice to make, talk to your mom or dad. They were kids once. They still remember. Have them help you decide what to do.

And what did my dad do about those chickens who were picking on one another? In order to protect the poor chicken who was all bloody, he put red plastic over all the windows in the chicken coop!

Why? Because when the sunlight filtered through the plastic-covered windows, *every* chicken looked red! There were none that appeared different and, therefore, vulnerable to the bullies.

Simple, huh? But oh-so-smart. We all have to do our best to protect our friends and those who are vulnerable to taunting and teasing. Good luck.

There is a girl in my class whose name is Phyllis. She is black. Another girl in my class is always gossiping. She always says to me, "Do you actually LIKE Phyllis?" I do, but when I say "yes" she is really mean and says "ew!" Should I tell Phyllis?

—Candice

What would the purpose be in telling Phyllis that someone is saying something mean about her? Would it make the other girl stop gossiping? No. Would it make Phyllis feel good about herself? No. Would it help the situation? Probably not. If you want to talk to someone, talk to the girl who is saying the mean things. Tell her that Phyllis is your friend and that you don't like hearing unkind things about her—and then don't listen to the cruel things anymore.

Too much talking—gossiping—about what "he" said and what "she" said will cause more problems than it will cure. It says in Proverbs 15:4, "Evil words crush the spirit."

We must be very careful what we say about others. We must control our tongues. "A big forest fire can be started with only a little flame. And the tongue is like a fire" (James 3:5–6). Once words are spoken they can never be taken back—they are already out of your mouth.

Apologizing is never as effective as not having said a

hurtful thing in the first place. Saying unkind things is like setting a fire that you won't be able to extinguish.

Has your mother or grandmother ever said to you, "If you can't say something nice, then don't say anything at all"? It's an old-fashioned cliché but it's still good advice.

I have a brother with Down's syndrome. It is hard to watch your brother struggle at something that is so easy for others. He is one of a kind. He can always make you laugh. I wouldn't trade my brother for anyone else because he is very special to me.

—Dulce

My favorite book of the Cedar River Daydreams series is Unheard Voices. *Like Ruth in the book, my sister is also hearing impaired. Some people treat her as though she has no feelings.*

—Aida, age 9

I'm having some of the problems Lexi had. I have a handicapped brother. I've moved a lot in my life. It's hard on me because people make fun of me and my brother at church and school.

—Cynthia

I don't have much time for people who tease others less fortunate than themselves. That tells me that the persons who do the teasing don't have much self-respect, compassion, kindness, or even common sense! It is *easy* (and childish) to hurt someone who is helpless to defend himself. It is *difficult* (but mature) to befriend such a person. Someone who teases the handicapped is announcing to the world, "Look at me, I am cruel, immature, and insensitive."

Just because some people at your school make fun of the handicapped doesn't mean you have to do the same. In fact, you might even be able to help turn the situation around. Read the next letter to understand what kind of a difference one person can make.

There is a boy in my class who's a dweeb. Naturally, everyone picked on him but I straightened up my act. It was hard to fight the peer pressure, but I did it! This boy was cautious of me at first because I was nice to him. I worried about having done things to him because I wouldn't have done those things to Jesus or anyone else. He was so hyped up that when I'd smile at him he'd tell me to "shut up." By the end of the year he had learned to trust me. I imagine it will take a while for him to become a real part of our class. He even traded school pictures with me. I was the first one. After that, almost the whole class traded with him. I'm glad I could make some kind of difference.

—Lyndsey, age 12

One person *can* make a difference! When you are tempted to go along with the crowd, remember that.

TWELVE

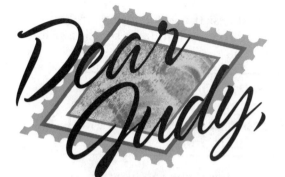

"My Friend and I Had a Terrible Fight..."

●●●●●●●●●

I've had a friend since grade school. We got in a fight because her boyfriend broke up with her and asked me out. I asked her if she still liked him. She said no, so I told the boy I would go out with him. We both agreed not to tell her for a while but she found out anyway. Now she won't talk to me. One morning at school we had a terrible fight and called each other awful names. She pushed me and I just walked away. We have not talked since then. I quit going to lunch with her and my other friends. I wrote her a note telling her that if she needed a friend I would be there for her. What should I do next? Should I try to be her friend or just give up?

—Netta

Friendships are precious and shouldn't be given up without some effort to repair the damage. Unfortunately, you did deceive your friend, whether you meant to or not. I realize that your intentions were good, but I'm sure your friend sees your efforts to keep your relationship with her former boyfriend secret as betrayal.

Put yourself in her shoes. If a boy had just broken up with you and she started to date him (and kept it a secret from you), how would you feel?

Imagine how good it would feel to be forgiven and have your friendship restored! Friendships are worth the effort to repair.

You were right to ask her if she still liked this boy, but you didn't go quite far enough. You should have told her you were interested in dating him yourself. She might not have liked it, but it would not have been such a stunning surprise to her if you'd been more forthright. It is much better to be "up front" about things than to keep secrets, which usually are found out anyway.

What would you have done if, when you told her you'd like to go out with her ex-boyfriend, she'd asked you not to? You might have gone out with him anyway. Or, you might have decided that this girl's friendship was worth more to you than a few dates with a boy. At least you would have had everything out in the open. Now you are left with the problem of untangling lies and deception.

It is good that you made the first effort to restore your friendship. I'd encourage you to try again. Perhaps an apology would help. If, however, after several tries, she doesn't respond, you may have to reconcile yourself to the fact that you've lost a friend.

I would hope the two of you could both forgive and forget what has gone on between you. Imagine how good it would feel to be forgiven and have your friendship restored! Think about the forgiveness God has shown to us. We've disappointed Him over and over again, and yet He still loves us. Incredible!

THIRTEEN

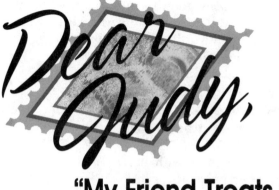

"My Friend Treats Me Like an Enemy..."

●●●●●●●●●

I have a friend who hates me, yet I pray for her a lot. She's always trying to find ways to make me mad. Can you help?

—Laura

I find it interesting that you call this person a "friend." She "hates" you and is always trying to find ways to make you mad. She doesn't sound like much of a friend to me.

Webster's New Collegiate Dictionary says that a friend is "one attached to another by esteem, respect, and affection . . . one not hostile; one not a foe." Does your friendship meet those criteria?

Still, it's great that you are praying for her. That is an appropriate reaction for any situation. It shows me that you are forgiving and generous. In fact, this reminds me of the verse in Matthew 5:3, "But I tell you, don't stand up against an evil person. If someone slaps you on the right cheek, then turn and let him slap the other cheek too."

When someone hurts us, our first inclination is to hurt them back, but Jesus tells us not to do that. Instead, He says we are to do even *more* good to the person who has hurt us! We are supposed to forgive those who hurt us and show them even greater love. I believe you are doing as Christ would have you do. Be patient with her.

It's a tough assignment, but the key to winning over an enemy is to show him or her even greater love.

Do you try to spend time with her even though she behaves this way? Then back off for a while. See if putting some space between the two of you helps. Do you share a table at lunch or walk to and from school together? Give yourself a little room. Walk home with others.

Perhaps she is jealous of you. Try to understand what makes her behave this way. That will make it easier for you to accept and understand her behavior—and maybe help to change it.

It may be that you will never really get along with this girl as well as you would like. Don't be discouraged. We can't please everyone all of the time. Maybe this is one of those people you will never please. All you can do is your best.

I saw that you wrote a note at the back of your book. It said that if I had problems that I should tell someone. Well, my best friend has been ignoring me. When I'd go up to her, she would move away from me. I told her that if she was going to treat me like that I didn't want to be her friend at all. Was that the right thing to do?

—Rhonda

That depends. Did you mean it? Are you really ready to give up your friendship with this girl forever?

I can understand your frustration. I would feel exactly the same way if my best friend began to ignore me. I'd be hurt, angry, confused, sad, and a dozen other painful emotions as well.

If my best friend did this to me, I would attempt to find out *why* she was acting that way. Perhaps I unintentionally hurt her feelings. If I did, I'd like to know so that I could apologize. Perhaps she heard that I'd said something bad about her (and I really hadn't). I'd like to know that, too, so I could tell her the truth. Do you see what I mean? I wouldn't throw away a friendship too quickly. I'd try to find out what has gone wrong so that I could repair the damage if possible.

Can you call her on the phone? Go to her house to talk to her? Write her a letter expressing your concern? Once you've made a big effort to reach her, it is up to her to respond to you. If she doesn't respond, then there is little more you can do.

FOURTEEN

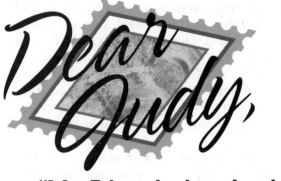

"My Friends Are Jealous..."
● ● ● ● ● ● ● ● ●

I'm pretty smart. Some kids are jealous of me and tell my friends lies. What would you suggest I do? I have prayed to God and things have changed a little. You had a great solution to Minda's jealousy of Lexi, maybe you have a solution for me.

—Tamara, age 12

It's often difficult to be seen as "the smart one." School is competitive anyway, and when you are identified as one of the brightest, it is easy to become the target of jealousy and envy.

The first thing you must remember is that your intelligence is a gift. Each of us has different gifts. Some can sing; others can play the piano. Some people are athletically inclined; others can paint marvelous pictures. Your intelligence does not make you more or less special than anyone else—just different.

I understand your predicament because I, too, did well in school. I was often teased when I didn't get a perfect score on a test or paper. People expected me to get good grades, but a few were obviously quite pleased if I didn't.

I have a hunch that occasionally you are tempted to pretend that you *don't* know some answers just to avoid the jealousy and teasing. I don't recommend you do that. Your intelligence is a gift for you to use and enjoy. On the other hand, it is important that you not flaunt that gift—don't show off or boast about how smart you are. Do your school-work to the best of your ability. Learn all you can. But don't remind others of all the good grades you earn. That's what modesty and humility are all about.

Though I got good grades, I was an athletic *disaster.* I didn't like running or competitive sports. My only poor grade in college was in an archery class. (It's a wonder that I didn't hurt someone with my bow and arrow!) And I certainly can't sing.

Your friends will have to discover their own gifts, the things they are best at. If necessary, help them by pointing out their strengths. When people have confidence in their own abilities, they don't have nearly as much need to put down the strengths and talents of others.

Surprise your tormentors. Fluster them with kindness.

It is the job of a Christian to be happy for those who have successes and to share the grief of those who have trouble. We're really all a community—a community of be-lievers. And when something good happens to one member of that community, it happens to all of us. At least that's the ideal way.

When someone comments about your good grades, compliment them on something special or unique they have achieved or that they do well. It's difficult to dislike someone who says nice things about you. Perhaps this will diffuse the jealousy and the lies.

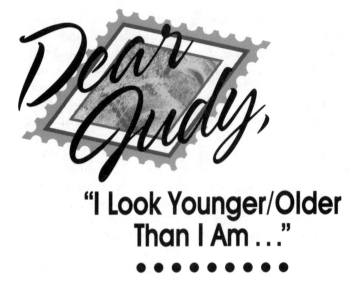

FIFTEEN

"I Look Younger/Older Than I Am..."

●●●●●●●●●

Some of my friends have already started their periods and their chests are bigger than mine! I feel so left out. I talked with my mom but she said just to wait and not worry. What should I do? Please help me; give me some advice.

—Lindsey

Time will fix all these problems. Some girls just develop more quickly than others. Each body has its own unique timetable. That's why you can't compare yourself to your friends. Some girls will appear fully developed by age twelve or even younger. Others don't "blossom" until they are closer to sixteen (or even older). Someday, you'll enjoy being different and unique, although it's hard to believe that right now. Just be patient, your body will "catch up."

I'm twelve and most girls my own age hate me because I look like I'm sixteen.

—Inez, age 12

I can sympathize with you. I was five feet seven inches tall in the fifth grade. When my group class picture was taken, I ended up on the floor *beside* the risers. I was too tall to stand *on* them and, if I stood in front, I'd block some of the other students! By the time I was an eighth grader, I was being asked what college I attended. Fortunately, by the time I was a senior, the other girls had caught up and I didn't feel so tall anymore!

Frankly, it's crummy to look so much older than your peers. For one thing, just when you really want to "blend in" and look like your friends, you begin to stand out—like the giant in "Jack and the Beanstalk." What's even worse is that people (strangers, teachers, sometimes even relatives) expect more of you because you look older than you really are. Then you hear things like, "You're too old to be doing that!"

It's wonderful, isn't it, how God made each of us special and distinct from everyone else?

It gets even more complicated when, as in your case, your friends begin to *resent* the way you look.

Your friends are jealous. Older boys are looking at you in a way they aren't noticing others your age. Your girl friends want that attention for themselves, that's all. You'll have to understand their jealousy—and be patient. Right now you are making the girls around you feel *insecure*. (And we all dislike that feeling!) But keep in mind that it is the other girls' problem, not yours. Don't let them make it your problem!

This is one situation that time will definitely cure. Soon they'll begin to develop as you already have. Your primary job right now is to maintain your poise. Don't get rattled by their harsh, childish words. (It's ironic, but when you get to be a mother or grandmother your friends will be competing to see which of you looks the *youngest*, not the oldest!)

Your true friends, the ones who know you as a person,

will like you for who you are, not how you look. As long as you can keep this problem in perspective, you can handle it. (And if it's any comfort, I'm sure you'll live through it. I did!)

SIXTEEN

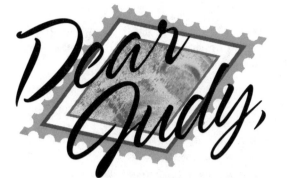

"I'm Glad God Doesn't Make Everyone Alike..."

● ● ● ● ● ● ● ● ●

I have some friends who have learning disabilities. They really are smart. They're no different than anyone else. They're special! I'm glad that God doesn't make everyone alike.

—Allison, age 11

I'm glad God doesn't make everyone alike too! What a dull, boring world this would be if we were all exactly the same. Still, all this variety God has given us creates responsibility. We must learn to accept others who are nothing like us physically, mentally, or even spiritually.

When we refuse to accept others who are different from us, several dreadful problems arise—racism, prejudice, intolerance, bigotry, class consciousness, feelings of superiority or inferiority, fear, and conflict. Yuk! What an ugly list!

As Christians, we must remember that God created *all* of us and we are equal in His sight. That means that we have no reason or excuse for looking down on someone if, for example, their skin is a different color or their physical abilities are impaired. *We are all equal!*

As Christians, it is our responsibility to find the good and the positive in every person and to focus on that, not the differences that might divide us.

I love your books soooooo much, they're so interesting; I have the whole collection. You would probably think that I wouldn't read your books, because I have a mostly-shaven head, and it's dyed black. Everyone calls me a punk-skinhead.

I just wanted to say your books interest me very much. I'm pretty sure they interest different types of people too, like me!

—Addie, age 14

A shaved head is certainly not common, but if under that shaved head is a generous, loving, and compassionate mind, great!

You do, however, make a statement with your looks. To most people, the look of a "punk-skinhead" states that, "I am a rebel. I don't follow the crowd. I don't respect authority. I want to stand out. I am brave and individualistic, perhaps even wild. I want people to be slightly afraid of me." Is that what you mean to say? If it is, then your look is working.

If, however, you are really shy, quiet, and struggling to find out exactly who you are as a person and you are using the dramatic look as a tool, then the look may be giving people the wrong impression about the kind of person you really are.

What a person is on the inside is far more important than what they look like on the outside.

God loves us all—the skinhead, the handicapped person in the wheelchair, the disabled veteran, the beautiful model, the child, the housewife.... And He loves us equally. We have no excuse to look down on some people and up to others. He doesn't.

What's more, He sees our hearts. He knows who is kind and loving, who is jealous and cruel. That's the part of us that we should make sure is dressed properly every day.

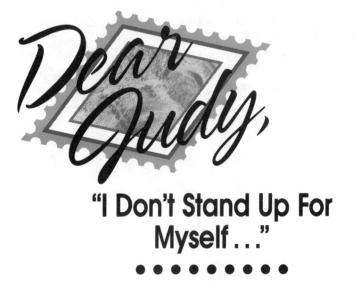

SEVENTEEN

"I Don't Stand Up For Myself..."

● ● ● ● ● ● ● ●

Your books are my favorites because Lexi stands up for herself and what she believes in. I can't do that at my school. I'm afraid if I did, I would have the entire school mad at me. I'd like to have Lexi's courage.

— Tabitha, age 13

A good deal of Lexi's "courage" is really *self-confidence.* She believes in what she says and does. She tries to do the good and right thing whenever she can. She's confident of her opinions and willing to stand up for them. That's the source of Lexi's bravery.

Self-confidence is something that must be built gradually over time. It starts when a child is in infancy. Do you notice mothers praising their children for little things? Baby's first unsteady steps or garbled words? Each time children are praised for something done well, they grow to have confidence in their actions. Gradually those actions become more bold, more sure.

Lexi is encouraged by her family to defend what is right

and oppose what is wrong. That's why Lexi in the Cedar River Daydreams books is able to take a stand against shop-lifting, homelessness, abuse, and racism, even though her opinion isn't always the popular one (especially with the Hi-Fives).

Don't worry—the world won't end if you stand up for yourself. In fact, it just might get better!

You can't change overnight and shouldn't even try. What you *can* do is pick an issue that is very, very important to you and let it be known how you feel about that one subject. When you discover that the world doesn't end if you stand up for yourself and for what you believe in, then perhaps you'll be ready (self-confident enough) to tackle another issue. This is all part of growing up.

I dislike conflict. I prefer to try to make everyone happy. But you *can't* make everyone happy all of the time— or even *part* of the time! So, when a controversial subject comes up, you have to be polite, pleasant, and firm. Don't be nasty to people who have an opinion different from yours. We live in a country where differences of opinion are encouraged and celebrated. You'll have to learn how to do this slowly—one step, one experience, one discussion at a time.

I think people could learn lots of lessons from the Cedar River Daydream books—like me, for instance. There is a girl in my class who was always asking me to call this boy for her. I did it but I didn't like it. Then I read the book about Lexi standing up to Minda and I said to myself, "Maybe I should do that too." When I refused to make the calls any longer she flipped and got so mad at me. Now we are friends again and she only calls me once or twice a day.

—Joanna, age 12

Good for you! You did exactly the right thing. You and

only you are in control of your life. Don't allow your friends to force you to do anything demeaning, improper, or uncomfortable. You were "brave" and it worked out fine.

Of course the girl was angry with you for refusing to do something for her! Babies are *furious* when they don't get their own way, too. But they get over it—and so did the girl you mentioned.

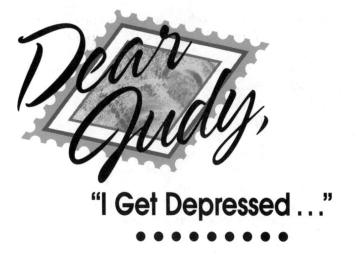

EIGHTEEN

"I Get Depressed..."

● ● ● ● ● ● ● ●

When I come home from school, I think too much about my problems. I need a way to keep from falling into deep depression. I read books.

—Deanna, age 11

I get depressed occasionally, but I guess most thirteen-year-old girls do from time to time.

—Nettie

There are ways to fight those "blue" feelings that wash over you once in a while. *Get busy.* Find something to distract you from whatever is bothering you. Visit a friend. Wash the dog. Volunteer to wash windows, mow grass, shop for groceries. Whatever you do, *don't sit there thinking about how awful you feel!*

As a little girl, I remember my mother putting me into the car for a drive. We'd look at the fields or stop at someone's house for a visit. She said that getting out of the house

79

made her feel better. Even as a child, it made me feel better too. That's what you have to do. Get out. Get distracted. Get better.

When you're feeling blue, you might have to force yourself to get up and do something. That's okay. Force yourself.

Another great way to fight off mild depression is with exercise. I assure you that I hate to exercise. I never really want to do it, but once I start I immediately begin to feel better. (There is actually a *chemical* reason for this—something about the brain creating endorphins or something.) I don't understand the reasons, but I know it works. Therefore, run, walk, jog, swim, bike, hike, dribble (a basketball), pump (iron), or do cartwheels. Just get moving.

I encourage my daughters (and just about everyone else who gets into a conversation about this with me) to journal. Get an empty notebook and a pen and start writing. Pour your emotions out onto paper. Tell that non-judgmental, non-critical piece of paper what's wrong. It's amazing how good it feels to get those feelings out of yourself and onto paper. What's more, when you go back to read what you've written, occasionally you realize that what's been upsetting you isn't such a big deal after all. (Sometimes it *is* a big deal, however, and that's when you need to seek more help.)

Sometimes depression is so serious that the above suggestions won't help. If you simply *can't* force yourself to get out of bed, if you cry or sleep too much, if you feel ill, if you don't want to spend time with your friends or do the things you used to love to do, then you may need professional help.

Everyone gets "down" occasionally but if it becomes chronic, then it is time to do something about it. Depression can lead to serious problems—misuse of alcohol, drugs, even suicide. There are medications that can be prescribed for depression. If you are suffering from depression, it's a good idea to go to a doctor for a check-up. After all, there might be a physical reason for your condition. Once you've been checked-out (and if everything is okay physically), counseling or therapy might be the next step—for you and perhaps for your family. There is no shame in asking for and seeking help. You'd probably be amazed at the number of people who have gone for counseling at one time or another. Besides, a therapist is duty-bound to keep what you tell him (or her) private. There is no reason for your friends or classmates to find out that you're going for help unless you choose to tell them.

TALK TO YOUR PARENTS. TELL THEM WHAT IS TROUBLING YOU. DO NOT DELAY. There are people who can help you. Let them know what is wrong so that they can help.

I'm involved in many activities such as jazz lessons, ballet lessons, organ lessons, art lessons, school sports, band, 4-H, and school choir. I don't have a lot of time for much else because I have so much practicing to do. Sometimes I just want to get away from it all. I've been considering running away—even for a little while. My friends aren't much help either. They act like I don't even exist. Sometimes I get so depressed over it all that I just cry and cry. I'd like to talk to my mom, but I think it would just make her worry. I feel so lonely, that no one cares. I've felt like that a lot lately and I don't know what to do about it. I come home from school feeling like this and no one's home because my parents work and I feel even worse.

—Yvonne

You *must* get some help! Don't delay any longer. It sounds to me as though you are *too* busy. It's great that you are involved in so many interesting activities, but you also need some time for yourself. You may be suffering from what is sometimes called "burn-out." You've put all your energy into your activities for too long without a rest and now you're worn out. You don't feel like doing anything at all anymore.

I can always tell when one of my daughters is suffering from burn-out. She gets stressed and exhausted. The best thing for her to do is sleep. Sometimes she'll sleep twelve hours, take an afternoon nap and go to bed early that night! But, after a quiet, restful weekend in which she can read, sleep, and soak in the tub, she feels great. She's no longer tired or stressed and she's ready to get back into action.

Can you give yourself a mini-vacation from some of your lessons and practice sessions? Can you use a Saturday or Sunday afternoon to just do some things for yourself? (You might give yourself a manicure, do your hair a new way, read all the books that have been piling up by your bed, or just nap.)

Running away isn't going to help your problems. In fact, that will create even *more* trouble for you. You will terrify your parents, put yourself in jeopardy, and do nothing to work out the troubles you'll have to face again when you return.

If you must "get away," ask to visit your grandparents or a cousin for the weekend. Visit a friend in another town. Maybe your mom would like a get-away too. Occasionally I tell my family I want to go on a "road trip." The girls roll their eyes and my husband smiles. On these little trips, we may not go more than 125 miles from home. (And that's not so far when you consider that our nearest fast-food restaurant is thirty-five miles away!) I look at things I usually don't take the time to visit. I like to stop at the Humane Society and pet the cats or go to a museum or store that I've heard of but have never visited. I come home refreshed. It seems to me you need a change of pace right now. We all do at some time or other.

Talk to your mother about your feelings and depression! I can't emphasize this enough. You think talking to her would make her worry? *Imagine how much she'd worry if you ran away!* Trust her. Let her help you. If it's hard to talk to her, show her this letter. Tell her this is how you feel. Ask her to help you. That's what moms are for.

I realize that it is difficult to come home to a quiet, empty house and that you probably feel worse than ever when you do. Therefore, change your habits. Study with a friend after school. Go to her house or have her come to yours. Go to the city library and study there. Perhaps there is a nursing home in your neighborhood or an elderly person who would love some company. Stop there to say hello. Brighten someone else's day and yours will be brighter too.

Your problems are not insurmountable. They can be managed, but please don't try to do it alone. There are people who love and care for you. You know who they are. Allow them to help you.

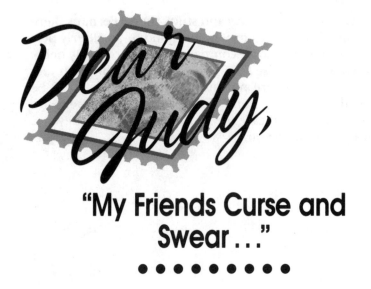

NINETEEN

"My Friends Curse and Swear..."

● ● ● ● ● ● ● ● ●

I love Cedar River Daydreams books. They always keep me on track. My friends curse. I like my friends but I don't like their cursing. When I read about Lexi and her friends, they keep me from cursing.

—Lisa, age 14

I think of myself as Lexi Leighton and try to make the same types of decisions she does. I am a Christian and go to a Christian school, but some of my friends swear and don't act like Christians. I faced the hard choice between keeping them as good friends or making other friends who are a better influence. After reading your books, I made my decision.

—Stormie

Sometimes people develop a habit of bad language. They use it so much and so often that they no longer even realize how it sounds. They have forgotten that God's name should be used in times of praise and thanksgiving, not anger or jest.

In the Ten Commandments, God says "You must not use the name of the Lord your God thoughtlessly. The Lord will punish anyone who is guilty and misuses his name" (Exodus 20:7).

Some of the most common expressions we hear include the name of God, but they are rarely spoken in a prayful fashion. Careless bantering about the name of God has become so commonplace that we've almost forgotten what it is we are saying. After all, it is *God* we are talking about— our heavenly Father, our Lord and Savior, the One who created us! When someone uses God's name in a curse or swear word, it indicates how that person really feels about God.

It is hard to have friends who curse. Can you say to them, "Don't say that around me, it makes me uncomfortable?" Can you tell them that it hurts you to hear the name of the God you love used like a swear word? Can you say, "Don't *do* that!" every time God's name is used in vain? It really depends on how comfortable you feel with your friends (and how they feel about you) when it comes to changing bad habits.

What you *do* can speak louder than what you say.

Frankly, some friends will make the effort for you, others will begin to ignore or dislike you. Perhaps you will decide that these kids aren't good for you to be around and you will break off the friendship. Just remember this—"Do not change yourselves to be like the people of this world. But be changed within by a new way of thinking. Then you will be able to know what is good and pleasing to God . . ." (Romans 12:2).

The one thing you *can* control is your own language. It's easy to slip into the careless habits of those people around you, but fight against it. Christianity needs to be your lifestyle. The way you live is important. What you *do* can speak as loudly as what you *say*.

TWENTY

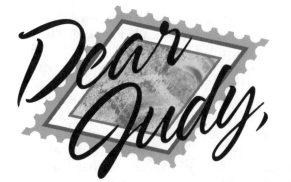

"Am I Hanging Out With a Bad Crowd?"

• • • • • • • • •

One of my friends is going through a very hard time. She is lying a lot. She's also stealing. My friends even say that she is a lesbian. What should I do?

—Marissa

Hmmm. . . . This is a tough one. Your friend is definitely showing signs of being in trouble. Do you know what is going on in her life right now that would cause her to rebel to the point of lying and stealing? Are there problems in her family? Is she hanging out with a bad crowd? Is she trying to get attention? Knowing *why* she's started this behavior would help you to understand what could be done to help her. Perhaps even a little concern and affection will assist her through this difficult stage.

I'd recommend that you talk this over with your mom. If she knows her, perhaps she can give you some clues as to why your friend is acting this way and what you can do or say to help her.

Talk to your friend. Let her know you care about her.

Tell her that you don't want her to get into trouble. En-courage her to go to her parents or pastor for help. There isn't much more you can do. God gave us all a free will. That is why we are able to choose to live any way we wish. Right now your friend is making some wrong choices. All you can do is convince her that you care about her and don't want to see her hurt herself.

Ignore the ugly rumor that your friends are spreading about this girl being a lesbian. That sounds to me like a cruel prank being played on a girl who already has a plate-ful of trouble. You shouldn't spread that rumor or even bring it up. It sounds like the result of too many idle tongues talking.

I just finished book #4, Journey to Nowhere. *I know some-body like Matt. He goes to my school and doesn't have many friends. The friends he does have are troublemakers. I know this boy better than most people. He's pretty nice. However, everybody is scared of him because his friends are good fighters. They got into a big fight at school and were suspended. I don't know what to do if my friends see me talking to this boy. I'm only twelve and in the sixth grade. This year is definitely the hardest.*

—Barbara

I realize that you like this boy (we'll call him "Matt") and that he may be a very nice guy. However, if Matt hangs out with troublemakers, then he may very well learn to be a troublemaker too. We are influenced by the people we spend time with. The Bible says it best—"Do not be fooled: 'Bad friends will ruin good habits'" (1 Corinthians 15:33). You don't want Matt to drag you down with him.

If you were my daughter, I would tell you to be polite and friendly to everyone (including Matt), but that you probably shouldn't take the friendship any further at this point. Your own reputation—as well as your value system, goals, and priorities—is built, in part, by the company you keep. Right now Matt sounds like he may be getting himself into trouble. You don't want that trouble for yourself.

Perhaps Matt will change. Hopefully, he will see that

the group he is associating with is hurting rather than help-ing him. Maybe he will decide to make new friends. Then you will have your opportunity to befriend him. But don't be disappointed if Matt never changes—some people don't.

People don't make radical life shifts easily or often. That type of change must come from within—and usually God is involved.

If your friend is telling you that you are "hanging with a bad crowd" listen to him. Ask yourself, honestly, if that is the truth. If it is, do something about it.

I have some friends who won't touch a book and are in to some pretty rotten stuff. Got any suggestions on how to get them to read something besides an album cover?

—Meg, age 12

Have you tried giving them some of your favorite books to read? Is there a particular topic that might interest them (music perhaps)? How about a tape or book by, or about, a Christian musician they've heard?

I don't know what you meant, but I don't like the sound of your friends being into "pretty rotten stuff." Sounds bad. You'd better ask yourself if you are actually influenc-ing your friends or if they are really influencing you. Be careful. You don't want that "rotten stuff" to rub off on you.

TWENTY-ONE

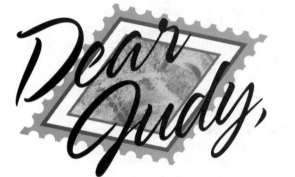

"If Your Friends Ask You to Do Drugs..."

● ● ● ● ● ● ● ● ●

This year I will be going to high school. It will be hard because a lot of people take drugs there. People will ask me but I don't want to take them.

—Beth

Former First Lady Nancy Reagan answered this question, *"Just say no!"* You don't have to explain yourself or give any excuses. Saying no is enough. If you are at a party or with a group of students who are pressuring you, leave. Tell those who try to intimidate you into doing something you don't want to do that you aren't into that sort of thing. Don't hesitate or beat around the bush. If you hem and haw, trying not to hurt someone's feelings, they will see you as weak. Just say no!

Remember—*you* are in control of your life and your body. Don't allow anyone to talk you into doing drugs or harming yourself in any way. Be strong on this. It's crazy to do drugs. Be firm. You won't regret it.

One of my readers figured out for herself what she was

comfortable doing when under pressure from her friends . . .

At my old school there was a group like the Hi-Five group. They were always making fun of people and doing dumb things. Even though I didn't like the girls and what they did, I wanted to be popular. When they asked me to do something stupid I remembered what Lexi had done. I told them I couldn't do what they asked me to do because I was a Christian.

—Lila

Just say "no"!

And there is really nothing more stupid than doing drugs. When it comes to drugs (and that includes alcohol), you must always do the brave, mature, and sensible thing— say no.

Some of my friends have had an experience or two using drugs. They got caught. Maybe if they'd read your book Fill My Empty Heart, *it would have helped them make the right decision.*

—Krystal, age 12½

I'm in a hospital because I have problems with drugs and alcohol, running away from home, and not going to school. I'm trying to get out of this mess.

—Devon

Getting caught isn't the worst of your problems if you do drugs—getting addicted is. Ruining your life is. Falling into destructive habits and patterns that will be difficult, if not impossible, to change is. Hurting your health permanently is.

I realize that many teenagers seem to think that alcohol is a "lesser" drug than marijuana, cocaine, speed, LSD, or heroine. It certainly is a more accessible drug, more commonly used, but that doesn't make it any less dangerous. Alcohol kills too.

You've all seen those TV ads telling you that if you drink, don't drive a car. That's because alcohol impairs your judgment, slows your reflexes, and makes you a general driving disaster. You could kill not only yourself but others—innocent people.

Drinking too much alcohol (bingeing) can result in alcohol poisoning. That happened to Peggy in *Lost and Found*. When you drink too much, the level of alcohol in your system gets too high and you may fall asleep and never wake up.

My husband is an attorney. He says people often insist they've only had "a couple of drinks," yet their blood alcohol level is over the .1 percent that is considered "legal" for drivers in this state. Alcohol makes you confused, forgetful, silly, weepy, obnoxious, sick, sloppy, gross, and a dozen other unpleasant things—it can also make you forget exactly how much of the stuff you've had to drink.

People who have a strong desire to "belong" often turn to alcohol because it makes them feel, at least for the moment, braver, prettier, stronger, more popular, less lonely. If you feel shy and awkward, alcohol might prop you up— for a few minutes. It's fake security, however. Once the alcohol is out of your system you'll feel just as you did before—only stupid and sick besides. Learn to deal head-on with whatever it is that troubles you—shyness, loneliness, insecurity—and you'll never need to depend on chemicals for any reason.

Refusing to take drugs is one way to avoid getting yourself into that "mess" to which my reader was referring. Stay away from drugs of all sorts. Life is difficult enough for teenagers. You don't need to take dangerous chemicals to make it worse. Just say no.

"That's not easy!" you say. "I don't know *how* to say no."

It's a simple two-letter word. Just say it. Don't make a big production out of it. You may even want to plan in advance how you will handle a situation in which you find yourself being offered alcohol or drugs. Write down your answers and practice saying them if necessary. Be prepared. That way you'll never be caught at a weak moment.

Just say no. *Always* say no.

PART II

Boys—Dating—Sex

● ● ● ● ● ● ● ●

You should know that your body is a temple for the
Holy Spirit. . . . You were bought by God for a price.
So honor God with your bodies.

1 Corinthians 6:19a, 20

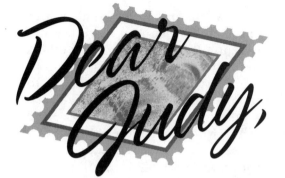

TWENTY-TWO

"Can Girls and Boys Be Just Friends?"

● ● ● ● ● ● ● ● ●

What if I have great friends that are boys (and not boyfriends)? People always tease me that I'm in love. I just hate it.

—Shelby

I think boys and girls can be friends without being "boyfriend" and "girl friend." My own daughters have friends (boys) that they have known since they were all in diapers. It would be sad if they couldn't remain friends as they grow up because someone insists that girls may only have girls as friends or that boys must be friends with only boys.

Some people are uncomfortable with the notion of boys and girls as friends because they have always viewed male/female relationships as sexual. That's why they tease you—because they doubt that boys and girls can share more than sexual attraction. Some people have never had deep, meaningful friendships with people of the opposite sex. Therefore, the idea may seem foreign and abnormal to them.

What's more, children and teenagers love to tease. Evidently you become upset when you are teased about this issue. Your response probably *invites* even more teasing! Instead of getting upset, just "grin and bear it." If others see that you aren't upset or flustered, the teasing will probably stop. Just in case, prepare a pleasant, witty answer to deflect the comments and continue to go about your business. As your friends mature, they will begin to see the value of having friendships with those of the opposite sex.

If you don't get upset, you will force the people teasing you to find a *new* target!

It is possible, of course, that at some point you may begin to see one of your male friends as *more* than just a casual friend. Perhaps one boy will stand out in a special way that makes you want to know him better and in a different way than all your other friends. It is then that a romance might begin.

That's fine too. I believe that people who fall in love and get married should do more than love each other. They should *like* each other as well. I'm a firm believer in the concept that you should marry a man (or in a man's case, a woman) who is his or her very best friend. Life isn't always easy. There is no better way to get through the rough spots than with a person who is your biggest cheerleader, your most compassionate listener, and your closest advisor—your *best friend*!

Don't let it get you down that others tease you. Just smile and let the comments bounce off you like rubber arrows off a bull's-eye!

TWENTY-THREE

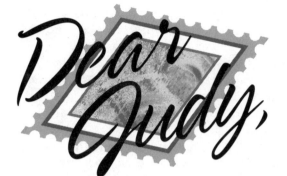

"All the Girls Are Fighting Over the New Boy in School..."

● ● ● ● ● ● ● ● ●

My friends have always turned to me with their problems. I would like to know if you would write a story about it. My problem is a little like your first book. A new boy moves to town and there is a "friendship war" about who he likes best and who he will go out with. This would help me out a lot.

—Alexandra

"Friendship wars" have been going on since kids started being kids. I can just picture your problem. Every girl in school is interested in the new boy (he's cute, he's interesting, he's *different* from the boys you are used to). Pretty soon the girls are getting mad at one another because of the amount of time or attention this new boy spends on each girl. After a while, the girls are all angry with one another, starting to say mean things behind one anothers' backs and generally having a miserable time. The new boy will pick one girl to like for a while, then go on to another and another, or he may decide that basketball (or hockey or softball) is more interesting than girls, anyway. Finally, the girls will start doing things together as friends should and the "war" will be over—until another new boy moves to town.

Here's the big question—*is the attention of a new boy in school worth risking a friendship over?* It's one thing to become serious about a man you'd like to marry. It's quite another to squabble over a boy you probably wouldn't want to marry even if you could!

Sure it's important to like and be liked by members of the opposite sex, but you'd have a lot easier time of it if everyone could keep things in perspective. Girls in grade school and high school are going to have lots of crushes on lots of boys. Seldom does one of these boys turn out to be "Mr. Right," the man they want to marry. So relax! Don't even bother getting into this silly "war." There really isn't much of a prize to be won.

Scrambling for attention from a boy isn't worth the tension it creates between you and your friends.

What you should do is be polite, pleasant, fun to be around. Don't chase this boy. Who knows? He might notice that you are different from the other girls who are vying for his attention and want to get to know you better!

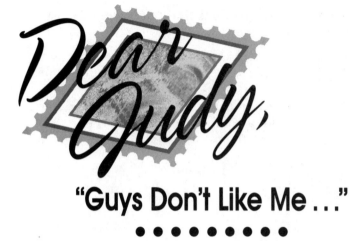

TWENTY-FOUR

"Guys Don't Like Me ..."

●●●●●●●●●

In my class there's one boy who all the girls (including me) like. I want him to like me so I try to just be myself. What he sees is what he gets. Some of the girls wear weird hairdos and do stupid things to impress him. He never pays attention to me but he always talks to them. What should I do?

—Collette, age 11

There really isn't much you can do. You can't *force* someone to talk to you. It sounds as though this boy is getting plenty of attention already. Why don't you focus your energy elsewhere? There must be other boys in your class. Do you like any of them?

I'm pleased that you decided to be yourself. That is a wise choice. No one really likes people who pretend to be something they are not. What's more, it's an uncomfortable charade—in a sense, you have to live a lie. Life is too complicated for that. Instead, be natural, be yourself, and be the best you know how to be.

Dear Judy,

Here are a few suggestions that might help you to be more natural around boys:

- Don't make them feel as if you want more than friendship (boys are often wary of that boyfriend/girl friend/romance stuff).
- Be friendly when you pass in the hall, (Say, "Nice shirt" or "You really did a good job giving your report.")
- Don't make fun of them—no one likes a person who taunts.
- Show interest in what the guys are doing. (You might find that you really enjoy football, classic cars, whatever . . .)

There is something else about your letter that I'd like to comment about. You are eleven years old. I realize, of course, that eleven-year-old girls like boys. At that age, girls are often more interested in boys than boys are interested in girls. So what if he's not talking to you now? What's the rush? Give him a few years to mature. By then he might realize how nice it is to know a girl who doesn't pretend to be someone she's not. Besides, all those others boys in your class will have grown up as well. Your tastes may have changed. You may no longer be interested in *him*.

When it comes to boy/girl relationships, the important thing is to *be yourself*.

I know it is hard, but if I could tell young women any single thing about boys it would be to relax and not rush into relationships or commitments. Don't worry (panic) like the next reader did. . . .

Silent Tears No More *gave me a lot of hope. I'm going into high school this fall and I've never dated anyone. All of my friends have, but I haven't. It doesn't seem as if guys like me. When Binky finally got asked out by Harry it gave me some hope.*

—Glenda, 9th grade

Please don't give up hope! You are barely at an age

where dating is appropriate. You haven't fallen behind in the boy scene—it sounds to me as though your friends have rushed ahead.

If you read the Cedar River Daydreams series, you know what a lovable, delightful, funny, tender, sweet person Binky McNaughton is. Yet Binky isn't flooded with boys asking her for dates. It took a *special person* (in Binky's case, Harry Cramer) to appreciate all of Binky's wonderful qualities. I firmly believe that there is a special person out there for you too.

As a teenager I always believed that God had a plan for my life. I trusted that when the time was right, I would meet the person that He had picked out for me. I really did turn that part of my life over to Him, and He did a far better job of picking out a husband for me than I would have for myself.

It takes patience and faith to get through these difficult teenage years—but you *will* make it. I did, and I didn't begin to date until I was sixteen.

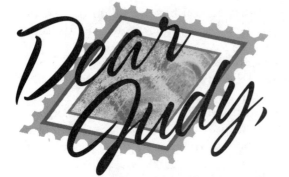

TWENTY-FIVE

Dear Judy,

"I'm Terribly Shy, Especially Around Boys..."

● ● ● ● ● ● ● ● ●

I'm a very shy person and have a hard time talking to guys older than me. What should I do?

—Irene

First of all, give yourself permission to be shy. Don't put yourself in situations in which you feel uncomfortable. Then it will be easier to work on getting over the shyness.

The only way to get over being shy is to practice. Perhaps you'll have to start by deciding to *smile* at a guy or two. That's it. No more. Once you are comfortable with that (and you realize that some of them will actually smile back), add a simple "hello" to that smile. When you feel comfortable with that, try, "Hello. How are you?" If you jump into being overtly friendly, you'll probably feel conspicuous and silly. Work into it slowly instead.

If your mind goes blank when you are talking to a guy, remember that showing interest in others by asking questions is a good way to break the ice, get to know someone and actually carry on a conversation as well. Ask questions. Let *them* do the talking!

Here are some examples of what you could say:

"Good game last night. How many points did you make?"

"How did you do on that chemistry test?"

"Great jacket. Where'd you get it?"

My suggestions might sound simple, but if you hit upon a subject of interest to someone, you can spark a fairly decent conversation. Then it is up to you to be a good *listener*.

If your mind goes blank when you're with a guy, *ask questions*. Then *he* has to do the talking!

I was never very comfortable with small-talk as a teen-ager, so I understand how you feel. Perhaps what you should do is let the guys talk first—and answer a question with a question. Tell them what you think about a topic you're discussing in class and then say, "How do you feel about it?"

Release from shyness comes one step at a time. Sometimes you will actually have to force yourself to be friendly. Just don't push yourself beyond limits with which you feel comfortable.

There is a seventeen-year-old guy who has a crush on me. I don't think I am very pretty. It makes me upset to think that anyone would think I am attractive. Men make me very shy, too, as well as some women. I am an all-around shy person. What do you do to get over shyness?

—Liz, twelfth grade

Why would you be upset that someone thinks you are attractive? That is a terrific compliment, one that many teenage girls would love to receive. Don't be upset—*enjoy* the fact that someone thinks you are special. After all, you *are* special. God made you—and only *one* of you. The Bible tells you in Psalm 139:13–14, "You [the Lord] made my whole being. You formed me in my mother's body. I praise you because you made me in an amazing and wonderful way. . . ." You are unique in the universe. Isn't it great that someone recognizes that? You will have to start accepting yourself as a wonderful, one-of-a-kind treasure before you can allow someone else to accept you.

Perhaps you just aren't ready for the "boy-girl thing" yet, and this boy's attention makes you nervous. If that's the case, that's okay. We all mature and develop at different rates. You might be alarmed by the attention now but will be ready and eager for it in a year or two.

People mature at different speeds and in their own personal ways. Give yourself some time. Perhaps you'll be one of those people who doesn't find anyone terribly appealing until—Wham! You fall head-over-heels in love with a guy you meet at a baseball game (or in college, or whatever).

Sometimes it helps to stop worrying about how uncomfortable we feel, and start to focus on the people around us.

I've gone into a room full of strangers and stood in the doorway thinking, *Now what? I don't know a soul. I feel so conspicuous. I wonder if my hair is all right. Maybe I should have worn a different dress. Everybody is talking to somebody but me. I feel terrible. I hate being shy. . . .* Pretty absorbed in myself, huh?

Other times, when I'm feeling strong and confident, I can go into a room full of strangers and think, *There's a lady with a pretty dress. I think I'll tell her how nice it is. I wonder where she got it,* or, *There's someone standing alone by the buffet table. She looks as alone as I feel. I'll go say hello to her. Maybe we'll strike up a conversation. I'd really like to meet some new people. . . .* Better attitude, right?

Don't be too hard on yourself. Take one area of your life and work on that. Perhaps that will mean smiling at people in the hallway at school (you don't have to say a word). And remember, other people are shy too. If you concentrate on others, you'll have less time to spend worrying about yourself.

TWENTY-SIX

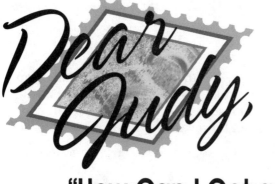

"How Can I Get a Boy to Like Me?"

● ● ● ● ● ● ● ●

I guess you could say I'm popular, but I really don't have any boyfriends. My mom says I'm pretty and that the boys are just shy!

—Anna, age 11

I'd believe my mom if I were you. You are only eleven. Boys your age are not very mature. Boys are usually a year or two, maybe even three, behind girls in both social and physical development at your age. You'll notice that the girls in your class are taller and more developed than their male classmates. You can't expect boys to be very brave around girls if the girls are several inches taller and seem so much older, can you? Give it time. Don't rush into adulthood too early. By senior high (when you really could be starting to date) you'll have plenty of boyfriends. I know you won't believe me—my own daughters don't when I say this—but, there is absolutely no hurry to have boyfriends. It's much better to have many friends, some of whom happen to be boys.

If I like a guy and he doesn't like me, how can I get him to like me?

—Karleen

As I've said before, you can't *force* someone to like you. That has to grow naturally out of mutual respect, attraction, and affection. There are certain things you can do to make yourself likeable, however.

- Are you always well-groomed (neat, clean, and looking your best)?
- Are you cheerful, pleasant, and fun to be around?
- Are you nice to people (friendly, interested in them, concerned about not hurting anyone's feelings)?
- Are you careful not to gossip or be petty?
- Are you a good sport?
- Are you interested in other people and not overly concerned with yourself (how you look, how people perceive you)?

If you work at all these things, it seems to me that it would be pretty hard not to like you!

You can't *force* someone to like you. That has to grow naturally out of mutual respect, attraction, and affection.

This one boy punches me, pokes me, undoes my bra, and teases me constantly. Does that mean anything special?

—Paula, age 13

Hmmm. . . . I imagine it does, but this guy is sending some pretty strange messages.

He's definitely interested in you (I don't know whether it's because he actually likes you or just likes tormenting you), but he is not very good at showing his interest. He is behaving in a clumsy, immature way. What he *is* revealing is that he is rude and thoughtless.

He wants your attention and apparently likes the response he gets when he pokes and punches you. I really don't approve of the bra thing and I'd tell him to "Stop it!" in no uncertain terms. When he's acting up in other ways, face him and say, "I'd like you a lot better if you wouldn't do those things. If you want my attention, just ask for it. I'd be glad to talk to you, but being poked in the back makes me angry."

Then, if he continues to be rude, you'll know that he's just a tease and really doesn't care how you feel . . . maybe. Thirteen-year-old boys are hard to figure out. The other side of the coin is that he may not know *how* to pay attention to you in other, more civilized ways. He might be crazy about you and is just so clumsy and inexperienced that he doesn't know what to do about it! (Fortunately, as guys get older they get better at showing and expressing their feelings toward members of the opposite sex.)

Ultimately, you will have to decide what he feels for you. If it is any comfort, men and women have been trying to figure each other out since Adam and Eve first walked the face of the earth. It's not easy—but at least it is an interesting challenge!

I go to church and believe in God just like Lexi does in your books. But in Fill My Empty Heart, *the book in which Binky and Harry date, I am more like Binky. I am eleven years old and there is a boy in my class that I like. Some girls say he likes me. I wondered if you could give me some tips about this.*

—Sasha, age 11

I would probably sell a lot of books if I could develop a foolproof method for romance and title it *How to Get a Boy to Like You.* Unfortunately, there is a little bit of chemistry, a dash of luck, and a pinch of mystery involved in this process—and I don't have the perfect formula.

Sometimes two people who seem perfectly matched don't get along at all. Other times, a couple who are so different from each other that it seems unlikely they will have anything in common fall madly in love.

If rumor has it that this boy likes you, he probably does.

If I were to formulate a list of suggestions as to "How to Get a Boy to Like You," here are a few of the things I'd mention:

1. Be friendly (but not pushy or silly).
2. Be genuine. (Don't say things you don't mean just because you think he might want to hear them.)
3. Smile.
4. Be pleasant, cheerful, and fun to be around. (Are you nice to people? Interested in them? Careful not to hurt anyone's feelings?)
5. Talk to him (but be careful not to gossip or be petty).
6. Be genuinely interested in his likes and dislikes. (Ask questions!)
7. Don't chase him. (That would only be embarrassing for both of you.)
8. Be well-groomed (neat, clean, and looking your best— yet not totally consumed with how you look or how people perceive you).
9. Be a good sport.
10. *Relax.* (Romance is not brain surgery. No one will die if this doesn't work out.)

I have an idea for your series Cedar River Daydreams. I'd like to read about a girl who is beautiful, smart, great to be around, and always ready to have fun. Her problem is that she really wants a guy to love her yet none of the guys are interested in her. Because of this she gets depressed and doesn't want to live anymore. If you could give me some insight into this problem I would appreciate it because that girl is me!

—Brenda

What's a beautiful, smart, fun girl to do when guys aren't interested in her?

First of all, don't be depressed about it! Give yourself some time. Girls who are too eager to have a boyfriend can scare boys off. Besides, if the "chemistry" isn't there and you and a guy don't click, it's just not going to happen anyway.

It's important to remember that you are a complete, interesting, vital human being whether you have a boyfriend or not. Enjoy your family and your girl friends (as Lexi does) and the rest will come at the right time.

Now, about the getting-depressed-and-not-wanting-to-live-anymore part—

When you are down, it may seem as though you will be feeling awful forever, but remember this, things *will* improve. If you do something truly stupid—like attempt suicide—you will be making a terrible, horrible, tragic mistake. I've heard interviews of people who've attempted suicide and failed. They admit being *glad* they failed. Why? Because once these individuals were on the road to recovery, their attitudes changed. They began to feel healthy again. Some met new mates. Others found a great job or received an award. Life went on and *it was better than they'd expected it to be.* Your life will too. No date (or the lack of one) is worth ending your life.

If you feel like committing suicide, *GET HELP!!!* Talk to a teacher, a parent, a pastor, an adult friend, an aunt, uncle, or grandparent. This is serious business. Depression can be controlled with counseling or medication. You don't have to feel like this, so *please* ask someone to help you.

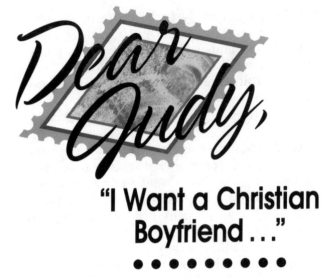

TWENTY-SEVEN

"I Want a Christian Boyfriend..."

●●●●●●●●●

I love Todd. If only I could meet a guy as perfect *as he is.* He's *great!*

—Sheila

I was hoping you could help me. I am fourteen years old and I want a Christian boyfriend. I know the Bible says that Christians shouldn't be unequally yoked. Is that for teens or for married and older people? I don't know what to do. I've prayed about it for a long time and nothing is happening.

—Cassie

The verse you are referring to is 2 Corinthians 6:14—"You are not the same as those who do not believe. So do not join yourselves to them. . . ."

It *is* very difficult to be married to someone who doesn't share your beliefs—especially something as *important* as your Christian faith. I would find my life very lonely and incomplete if my husband did not share my faith in God.

Even when a couple is dating, it is definitely more comfortable to share similar views about life. If you and the boy (or boys) you date have the same attitudes and belief systems—based on Christianity—then decisions about experimentation with things such as cigarettes, alcohol, drugs, and premarital sex will be "non-issues."

You might take that verse in the Bible—the one about being unequally yoked—as a reminder when you are beginning to date seriously (hoping to find the man with whom you'd like to spend the rest of your life), that you look for more than physical and intellectual compatibility. Spiritual compatibility is just as important for a long and happy married life.

It's easy to fall in love. It's harder to stay in love—unless you share all of the things that matter most.

But what you really want now is an answer to the question—Where do I *find* Christian boys? Church, Bible camp, youth groups, and youth rallies are the most obvious places. Of course, if every girl ran around at each of those events hoping to snare a boyfriend and were disappointed if she didn't, that would take most of the fun out of the event!

It's good that you've prayed about this, but you still sound very impatient. Now that you have asked God to help you, *quit worrying about it!* He heard you. He knows what you want (and what you need). He'll take care of it. Turn this issue over to Him. God knows things we don't. Perhaps at fourteen you aren't *ready* for a boyfriend yet (even though you feel *very* ready). Trust that when the time and circumstances are right, you will get your answer.

Does that sound hard? Especially since all your girl friends are beginning to date? Maybe it is. But if you've really turned this over to Him, you should be able to lean back and relax. God is willing to be more generous to us than we would ever be to ourselves. Let Him.

Dear Judy,

Enjoy your life, your girl friends, your family. Go places and attend functions that please you. Someday you will meet someone who enjoys the same things you do.

There aren't any boys like Todd! I know three Christian boys—Hal, Dave, and Bryce. Dave is worse than any "secular" boy. You should hear his mouth. Hal hangs around with him and is getting bad. They tease me. I'm like Lexi, I have a nickname—"Miss Perfect." If I do something like have an overdue book they have a cow! Bryce is the best but he is a smart-mouth and rude to teachers.

I like this kid named Jon. He is really nice and doesn't hang around in any "Hi-Five" group. (Neither do I. They make too much fun of everyone and can be snobs at times. Even so, they're nice when they're not together as a group.)

Jon's nicer than any of the Christian kids I know. He doesn't treat anyone like dirt.

—Geena, age 13

Saying you are a Christian and actually *being* one can be two entirely different things. True Christianity bubbles out from the core of you, influencing the way you believe, talk, and act. The three "Christian" boys you've described sound like they have a lot to learn—and need to examine their faith.

Perhaps you assume they are Christians because they come from families who attend church and have parents who profess to be Christians. Just because a parent is a Christian does not guarantee that his or her children will automatically be Christians too. Christianity is not inherited like blue eyes and blond hair. It is a decision, a leap of faith, and every person must make it alone. Lots of people *say* they are Christians (or at least go to church every single Sunday), but only God knows what is in their hearts.

I'm glad your friend Jon is nice. Maybe you should invite him to attend a church youth function. He might really like it.

Todd is exactly the type of guy I want. I really like a boy at school, but does he like me? I'm too shy to find out. During recess, he asked me to hold his sports bottle while he pushed the merry-go-round. Do you have any tips, suggestions, or anything else?

—Rhoda, age 11

The sports-bottle thing sounds promising to me! Whatever you are doing must be all right. Don't expect *too* much from him, however. After all, if he's only eleven, trusting you with his possessions might be as big a compliment as you will get from him!

Don't worry too much about attracting boys. Don't rush what is bound to happen anyway. Give yourself time to grow into a terrific teenager. Then when the really appropriate time for boy/girl relationships comes, you'll be prepared in all the important ways—with maturity, common sense, self-esteem, moral values.

Relax and enjoy right *now*. Hold the sports bottle if you wish, but don't try to hurry on to the next level of boy/girl relationships. It will come when the time is right.

TWENTY-EIGHT

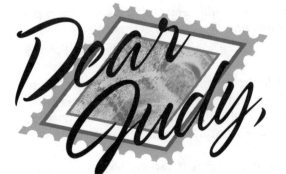

"My Parents Don't Know About My Boyfriend..."

• • • • • • • • •

I've got one problem. I have a boyfriend. He is our preacher's son. He asked me to go out with him. My parents don't even know I like him. I am only 11½, but I really like him! I feel better now that I've got that out. I was wondering if you would write back and give me some advice.

—Savannah

Sorry, but I don't like the idea of keeping secrets from your parents. It's okay to like a boy and not tell *everyone* about it, but once you start to consider dating you'd better let your parents into your life.

It sounds as though you aren't comfortable with your situation either. Look at what you wrote—"I feel better now that I've got that out." Secrecy and deception aren't fun burdens to carry.

He asked you to "go out" with him. What exactly does that mean? Does he want you to go as part of a group to a church or school function he will be attending? That might be okay with your parents. Or does he want to be alone with you at an unsupervised function? I'd guess your parents will say "no way" to that. Please realize that you two can be friends even if you don't tie yourselves exclusively to each other.

Your parents should be an important part of your dating life. They can offer you support, advice, and a listening ear.

Activities that used to be high school territory—dating, boy/girl relationships, parties, steadies, etc.—have now filtered into the lower and middle grades. Frankly, I think there's too much emphasis on couples and too little encouragement to have a broader range of both male and female friends.

You have your entire life to look for the perfect mate, but there are only a few years to have the fun that only kids can have. Do that now. Otherwise, you may later regret having tried to grow up too fast.

TWENTY-NINE

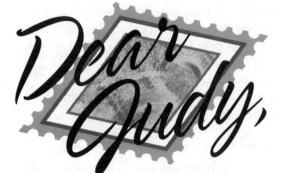

"My Boyfriend Doesn't Get Along With My Family ..."

● ● ● ● ● ● ● ● ●

My brother acts like a nerd. When my boyfriend calls or comes over to my house, my brother shows off and my boyfriend doesn't like it. I don't know if I should dump my boyfriend because he doesn't like my brother, or if my boyfriend and I should ignore his childish stunts.

—Edith

Why do you want to hang around with a guy who isn't mature enough to ignore your brother when he's goofing off? It appears that your brother is trying to *impress* your boyfriend (and not doing a very good job of it). Why don't you and your boyfriend try spending a few minutes talking to your brother or including him in whatever you are doing. Perhaps he'll act less obnoxious when he gets some attention.

I'd worry about your brother before I'd be concerned about your boyfriend. After all, this boyfriend may not be in your life for more than a few weeks or months. Your brother is your brother forever.

If things get really bad, talk to your mom or dad. Enlist their help. Perhaps they'll distract your brother or make him behave more like a human being. Parents like to keep peace in the family too, you know.

THIRTY

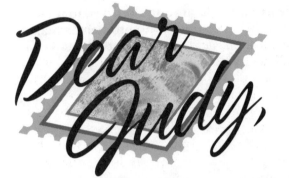

"My Parents Won't Let Me Date Until I'm 16!"

● ● ● ● ● ● ● ●

My parents won't let me go out! I've heard them say that they don't want me to go anywhere with a boy unchaperoned. They don't understand that going out is holding hands and being friends. I can't go out until I'm sixteen! *Do you know how I can change their minds? I love them a lot, but they're the strictest parents in the whole junior high!*

—Pamela, age 13

My parents think I'm too young for a boyfriend. All my friends have one. . . . . I am twelve years old and in sixth grade.

—Jocelyn

I am thirteen and have a boyfriend. We have only been going together for eight weeks. My friends get mad at me because I talk about him all the time. I am not allowed to date until I am sixteen.

—Tenneille

What, exactly, does it mean to have a *boyfriend*? Does it mean to know and like a boy who knows and likes you? That's okay in sixth grade, I think.

Or does it mean to have an exclusive relationship with one guy that involves a high level of intimacy, which includes a lot of time alone together? That's *not* appropriate for sixth grade and is even questionable for older kids. You may be setting yourself up for problems later.

The more time a couple spends alone together, the more likely they are to occupy that time kissing, hugging, etc. And once you start that, it takes more and more of the same to satisfy you each time you are together. One thing *does* lead to another and eventually you may be into some very intimate activities including petting and sexual intercourse.

What does "going out" really mean? If it means being friends, I can handle that. That's fine for young teens. My definition of "going out," however, is dating. Having a boy come to the house, picking up a girl to do a special activity such as bowling, golfing, etc. Being a couple.

Once you have a good idea of what it is you actually want to do, you will have to sit down with your parents and decide what you will be able to do and at what age you can do it!

Parents aren't monsters. Talk to them. Tell them how you feel. . . . Their goal is to do what is best for you.

It is not my place to tell you how old you must be before you can date. Nor is it my place to second-guess your parents. That is a family decision that you must make together.

Talk to your parents. Tell them how you feel. Ask them questions if you feel it's necessary. Then willingly go along with their rules. They are really trying to do what is best for you.

Here's a tip—often parents don't want their young teens dating regularly, but sometimes, for a special occasion such as a homecoming football game, they might agree to let you go with that boy you like so much. All you can do is ask. And if they say yes, then go, enjoy the evening, and be home at exactly the time they tell you to be (or earlier, if you really want to please them). If they say no, don't pout. Accept the decision cheerfully, knowing that your response indicates your maturity and may influence them the next time a special occasion arises.

THIRTY-ONE

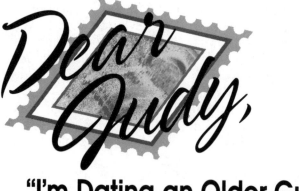

"I'm Dating an Older Guy..."

● ● ● ● ● ● ● ● ●

I really like this guy, but he's six years older than me. I think he likes me, but I am not sure.

—Ashleigh, age 12

I was wondering if dating a guy who is older than me makes a difference?

—Jamey

My answer depends upon how old *you* are. If a thirty-year-old woman dates a thirty-six-year-old man, their ages don't matter very much. Both are mature adults. However, if a twelve-year-old wants to date an eighteen-year-old (or someone fifteen is interested in someone twenty-one) then I think age matters a great deal.

There is a big difference in the maturity and experience levels of twelve- and eighteen-year-olds. (I know when my daughters were twelve they didn't believe me, and you probably won't like to hear it either, but it *is* true.)

I don't think teenagers should date anyone who is as much as six years older than themselves. In fact, I even wonder what is *wrong* with the eighteen- or twenty- or twenty-four-year-old who *wants* to date someone so much younger. Won't girls their own age have anything to do with them? Why? Sounds suspicious to me.

I'd recommend that you think things through very carefully before you do something you might regret later— and that includes seeing guys who are so much older and more experienced.

It may seem as though you'll never meet a guy who is just right for you, but have patience. It's not difficult to find boyfriends or to marry. What is important is to find the *right* person, the one you can comfortably and happily live with for the rest of your life.

THIRTY-TWO

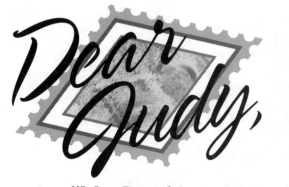

"My Boyfriend Isn't Very Affectionate..."

● ● ● ● ● ● ● ● ●

My boyfriend is always busy. When we're together we just act like friends. I know he likes me and I definitely like him, but we never show it. What should I do?

—Ella

Sounds okay to me. Maybe your boyfriend is *uncomfortable* with big displays of affection. If he likes you, you like him, and you enjoy being together, it appears to be a good arrangement.

Too much coziness in public isn't a good idea anyway. It makes the people around you feel uncomfortable and shows that you don't have much consideration for others.

If you *have* to do something, send him a funny card in the mail, one that reminds you of a humorous moment or laughter you've shared. Give him bright, I'm-happy-to-see-you smiles.

Be patient. When you are both comfortable with your friendship, he'll learn to be more outgoing.

THIRTY-THREE

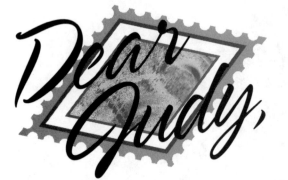

"Do Todd and Lexi Ever Kiss?"

● ● ● ● ● ● ● ● ●

Lexi's relationship with Todd made me realize that my relationships with my male friends aren't as strange as everyone says. There are three or four boys in my seventh grade class that I can talk to. I'm glad to know boys and girls can just be friends. For this, I thank you.

—Lynda

I love the kind of relationship Todd and Lexi have. I long for that kind of relationship with a guy! I especially like how comfortable Todd and Lexi are with each other. They are so open with each other. They are more best friends than boyfriend and girl friend. I think that is the best kind of relationship to have. Another thing I like is that they're not always together and dependent on each other. They both have other friends, and although they like to spend time together, they don't have their hands all over each other. (Peggy and Chad were like that. You know where that led them!) Listen to me! I'm talking as if Peggy, Todd, Chad, and Lexi are real! I'd like to believe that they are because I look to Todd and Lexi as role models.

—Shawna, age 14

I don't understand how Todd and Lexi can be boyfriend and girl friend without having any romance. It seems like they're just good friends. They never say "I love you" and they never seem to kiss. I don't understand. With all my relationships, it's been "love" more than "good friends."

—Trina

After reading all of the Cedar River Daydreams books, there is only one thing I would want to change. I'd like Lexi and Todd to be more romantically involved. My friend and I are always hoping they will kiss. Todd has kissed her nose and her forehead, but never have they really *kissed, you know.*

—Sabrina, age 13

Will you ever have Todd and Lexi get married? That would be really be neat. They belong together. I wish I could have a relationship like they do. It sounds pretty cool. Will Todd and Lexi every say "I love you?" Just curious.

—Janel

I would like to know if Lexi and Todd are every going to kiss? If not, why?

—Riley, age 14

I know that many are waiting for Todd and Lexi to *really* kiss (none of that friendly peck-on-the-cheek stuff they usually do). Frankly, I've been waiting for it too! But Todd and Lexi just aren't in to that yet.

When I was in high school, most couples either dated alone or with one other couple. Once you were part of a couple, you spent a lot of time alone together.

Now many teenagers spend their time together in larger groups—at one another's homes, shooting hoops, driving around, going to the mall, or even going out on actual dates that involve bowling or going out for pizza. They are still couples, but now, instead of going out alone, they often go out with five or six of their friends. It's the way many teenagers function in the 90's.

There's a lot less pressure to do the things couples normally do (kissing, necking, whatever) if you are part of a larger group. Not only that, it's actually more *fun*.

By hanging out in groups instead of pairing off, there is more time for real friendship and understanding to develop between members of the opposite sex.

That's the pattern Lexi and her friends at Cedar River have fallen into—they are together in an ever-changing mix of kids, depending on who is available and free.

In part, that is why there isn't much romantic interaction between Lexi and Todd. The other reason is that in my writing I've chosen to emphasize the importance of *friendship* and *relationship* over that of romance. Todd and Lexi do kiss. (If you read closely you can catch them at it once in a while.) But it is usually a friendly rather than a passionate sort of kiss—the kind of kiss that's healthiest for teenagers.

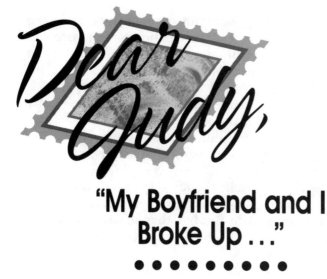

THIRTY-FOUR

"My Boyfriend and I Broke Up..."

● ● ● ● ● ● ● ● ●

I've had some problems with my boyfriend that I just can't go to my parents about. I know you are very busy, but if you could give me some advice I would really like it.

We broke up but then he wanted to try again! I told him no, so he started dating one of my best friends. Whenever I see them together he thinks I should act normally. He doesn't see that I'm hurt. We have become friends again, but I want more. I'd like to date him again! I'm confused about my feelings for him. First I want to go out with him and then I don't. It's so hard!

—Marie

It *does* hurt to see an ex-boyfriend with another girl. I can understand why it would be difficult to "act normally" when you see them together. However, you can't have it both ways. You didn't want to date him and told him so— you really didn't expect that he'd never go out again, did you?

It appears that the first thing you must do is make up your own mind.

Occasionally *wanting* something is more fun than *having* it. Things you *can't* have look very enticing—but once you actually *get* those very things, you might lose interest in them. That's called being "fickle." This means being indecisive, wishy-washy, unpredictable, and uncertain. It's not a very nice trait in one's personality, and it is certainly a hard characteristic for others to understand or tolerate.

Ask yourself some questions. Do you want this boy because you care for him and miss him, or because your best friend has him?

Be honest with yourself. If your answer is because your best friend has him, then stop thinking about him and let it go. You want to be with this boy for the wrong reasons, and you are only wasting time and hurting yourself and others in the process.

If your answer is that you care about him, then you must first consider your girl friend's feelings. She'll be hurt and angry if you try to interfere with the relationship she now has with this boy. (What kind of friend are *you*?)

You'll also have to admit you made a mistake and acknowledge your feelings of confusion and that you've messed up.

Discover how to learn from the bad times as well as the good ones. Look for the positive in every situation. Once you begin to find it, you'll be all right.

There is something else you must realize about this situation. You may have already blown it with this guy. He may not want you back. You've disappointed him before. He might not want to bother with you anymore. He may really like the girl he's dating now.

Then what happens?

Accept it. Don't get angry with the boy or his new girl friend. This is a situation of your own making. Take responsibility for what's happened. Learn from your mistakes. Your life isn't over. You are wiser and smarter now.

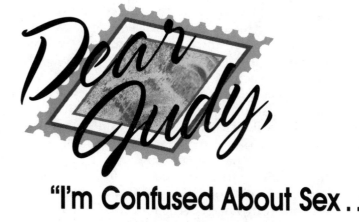

THIRTY-FIVE

"I'm Confused About Sex..."

● ● ● ● ● ● ● ● ●

I'm wondering if there is going to be any romance between Lexi and Todd. I haven't heard of many Christian books that involve teenage romance. I don't understand why some people act as if the Bible says that dating or kissing and hugging between two teenagers of the opposite sex is a sin. It isn't like they are having pre-marital sex or anything.

—Noele

I love romance books but I hate books that go into detail about people making out and stuff like that. It makes me wonder what some of those authors are thinking about. People complain that there are too many teenage girls getting pregnant, but they talk about it in their books.

—Olivia

Kissing and hugging aren't wrong. In fact, they are both rather nice activities—in the right time and place. Parents don't encourage their children in these areas because they know very well (from their own teenage years) that kids will discover soon enough just how nice kissing and hugging can be. What worries most parents is the *age* at which this type of activity starts and the *frequency and intensity* of these same activities.

Each teenager has to draw a line that he or she will not cross in a dating relationship. Choose friends (both boys and girls) who have similar interests and values. Always remember that God is willing to help you through this confusing, sometimes rocky part of your life too.

He *wants* you to be happy. He *wants* you to have a life-partner. He wants more good things for you than you could even imagine for yourself. Tell Him, "God, I'm really confused by this dating and sex stuff. Help me find the person who is exactly right for me, the one you have picked out for me. And help me not to make any mistakes along the way." Once you've done that, calm down. Your life is in good hands. He'll take care of you.

THIRTY-SIX

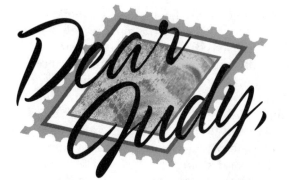

"Why Do I Feel So Pressured to Have Sex?"

● ● ● ● ● ● ● ● ●

Can I ask your advice? Boys can be such problems. Why do I feel so pressured to have sex with them? Some have asked me to and some haven't, but I feel that the only reason they like me is because of sex. I know I don't want to do it and that I can say no. I still feel used and it is degrading. I'm so confused. I just had to get some things off my chest. Whether you know it or not, you've helped me.

—Miki, age 14

There are probably several reasons you feel so pressured. One is the message that our society (through television, movies, magazines) is sending to its teens. If you believed everything you saw on TV, you'd think that every couple in America spent a large portion of their day thinking about or having sexual relationships. Teenage magazines are always giving advice on beauty, boys, and what else? Sex. Even though these aren't *true* pictures of American life, after we see them long enough, we begin to believe they represent the truth. Then we begin to wonder, *if these sexy people are the norm, and I'm not doing* any *of the things they are doing, then what's wrong with me?* That's pressure!

A second reason you may feel such stress is *hormones.* Teenagers are naturally interested in and curious about sex. Your body is changing, you're feeling things you haven't experienced before. The boys you know are going through similar changes. So, naturally, sex is on your mind more than it has ever been before. That is normal.

Another reason you may feel as you do is that you hear the line, "Everybody else is doing it," and you believe it. Unfortunately, some teenagers *are* sexually active. Others may talk like they are, but really aren't. Everyone is buckling under to the *untrue* idea that if they aren't sexually active they are missing something special. Peer pressure can make teenagers do all sorts of things they wouldn't normally do if they were using the "common sense" part of their brain rather than the "I-want-to-be-like-everyone-else" portion of their gray matter.

Don't do anything you will regret later. Sex is serious business. It is *adult* business. Once you start experimenting with your body, you will discover a multitude of new questions, problems, and challenges that you haven't even considered yet. You can get pregnant. You can contract diseases such as acquired immune deficiency syndrome (AIDS), chlamydia, herpes, syphilis, gonorrhea, and genital warts. You will lose your self-esteem. There is a good reason God wants us to have sex only inside a loving marriage relationship. His rules are for our protection, not punishment.

I'm glad that you already know that you don't want to do this and that you have the freedom and ability to say no. That's a positive and mature attitude. Keep it up.

Sex between a married couple who love and are devoted to each other can be one of the greatest experiences in the world. This is true for several reasons. Frankly, sex takes practice. You aren't great at it the first time or even the second. Inside a marriage relationship, you have the time, love, and freedom to learn and to enjoy what is right for your partner. What's more, sex is always better when there is commitment and love involved—the kind of commitment and love that brings one to the altar to speak marriage vows, not merely the kind of pledge that involves exchanging class rings and promises that can't realistically be kept.

Sometimes the best things in life are those things for which you have to wait. Sex is one of them.

An unmarried couple who feels pressured by either hormones or peer pressure into doing something neither is ready for can be an unmitigated disaster. I wish for you the best option—intimacy inside the bonds of love and marriage.

I have a very big problem. In the back of your books it says to talk to my parents, a pastor, or a trusted adult. But I cannot bring myself to tell my parents. . . . I used to go to a counselor, but we didn't get along. I was wondering if you had some ideas of who I could talk to. It's not that I'm pregnant, but it's sort of close, so unless I tell my parents they'll never find out. I feel so guilty about not being able to tell them.

—Ramona, age 13

It sounds to me like you are playing with fire and if you aren't careful, you'll get burned. Sexual activity is a funny thing—it's like a snowball that picks up momentum as it rolls down a mountain; by the time it reaches the bottom, it can cause a real avalanche.

You sound as though you really do need to talk to someone, and I'd encourage you to try your parents. It will be hard, I know, but they love you—more than you realize. Give them a chance. If school is in session, maybe the school counselor could help, or perhaps a teacher, your aunt, or an older cousin. But first, try your parents. You'll find that your mom and dad have an amazing capacity for love and understanding.

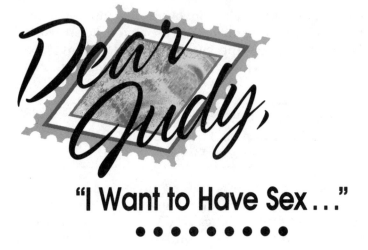

THIRTY-SEVEN

Dear Judy,

"I Want to Have Sex..."

●●●●●●●●●

Last night my parents and I got into a fight over my boyfriend. They told me I couldn't see him anymore. It isn't right for them to do this to me! He means a great deal to me and I don't want him out of my life.

The reason he means so much to me is because I had sex with him. Everyone tells me premarital sex is wrong and my church has always taught me to be against it but, to be honest, I don't believe it's all that wrong. I don't want to wait for marriage. I don't even want to get married, because the divorce rate is so high.

I know what I'm doing is unsafe and immature, but I really don't care. I suppose I should have some self-respect, but I really don't see it as a big deal. Life is so confusing. I've tried to talk about my feelings with my mom, but she doesn't know all the details of my life or what my boyfriend and I have done together.

—Karla

You sound bitter, confused, angry, and very low on self-esteem. Have you asked yourself what's caused this emotional crisis in your life?

Is it because you've been lying to your parents? Going against your church's teachings and God's rules for your life? Doing things that in your heart you know aren't good for you?

Having sex with your boyfriend hasn't made you any happier. It has only alienated you from your parents, forced you to keep secrets, and made you defensive about what you've done.

Since you've already come to this point in your life, the question is: *Now what?*

We can't put our lives into reverse and go backward to relive and repair some of our mistakes. The mistakes are made. Your virginity is lost. You can't regain it.

You *can,* however, start fresh, putting the past behind you, viewing the future as a clean slate with no marks upon it. That's what repentance is all about—admitting that you've goofed up (*sinned*), made mistakes, botched things, and asking God to forgive you for what you've done wrong. The second part of repentance is changing your life so you don't make those same mistakes all over again.

Talk to God about your life. Tell Him what's gone wrong. You may think this situation is something you can handle on your own but it's not. You've run out of self-esteem. You're confused. You're being self-destructive. Ask for His forgiveness and the opportunity to start anew.

God promises you this in Scripture: "But the evil person might stop doing all the sins he has done. And he might obey all my rules and do what is fair and right. Then he will surely live. He will not die. His sins will be forgotten. Now he does what is right. So he will live. I do not really want the evil person to die, says the Lord God. I want him to stop his bad ways and live" (Ezekiel 18:21–23).

One of the most astounding (of an unending list of astounding things) aspects of God is His generous willingness to forgive us when we do something wrong. He is *willing* and *able* to wipe the slate clean where our mistakes are concerned. God not only *forgives* but He also *forgets.*

You obviously aren't happy traveling the path that you are currently on. You feel crummy about yourself. You're confused. Take a break from what you've gotten into. Give God a chance.

Even though you've made some not-so-great choices up until now, you can, with God's help, start fresh in your life.

If you are honest with yourself you would have to admit that premarital sex hasn't helped you any. Tell your boyfriend that even though you've had sex in the past, you don't want to do it anymore. It doesn't mean you don't love him. It just means that you need to get your self-esteem back, to regain control of your life. If he doesn't agree with you and doesn't want to help you pull yourself together, that will tell you how much (or how little) he values you (your mind, your personality—not just your body) in the first place.

Here are some reasons a teenager might give for not wanting to have sex before marriage.

- I'm not ready.
- I don't want to have any regrets later.
- Everybody is *not* doing it.
- I'm a human, not an animal; I can control my urges.
- I'm saving myself for the person I marry.
- If this boy really loved (and respected) me, he wouldn't ask me to do this.
- I respect *myself.* I have nothing to prove by doing this.
- God says it's not a good idea and He knows best.
- I don't want to disappoint my parents.
- It goes against my values.
- This boy only likes sex, he doesn't even care about *me.*
- I don't want AIDS, herpes, syphilis, gonorreah, genital warts, or any of the other junk passed around this way.
- I'm still a teenager. I don't need this emotional baggage in my life.
- It would make me *lose* popularity and respect from my friends and peers.
- It is an act I can't undo. I'll never be a virgin again.

- I don't want to have a baby, and no birth-control method is one hundred percent foolproof.
- Love isn't sex and sex isn't necessarily love.
- When I do it, I want it to be special—not a cheap thrill in the back of a car.

Make your own list. You'll have more to add. If you really look at them closely, there's a lot more in favor of waiting to have sex than rushing into it for all the wrong reasons.

What I'm advising you to do isn't easy. I'd recommend that you get some help to work through this. You've tried to talk to your mom in the past—try again. And this time, tell her the *whole* truth. Tell her that you're feeling confused and sad. Ask her to help you find a counselor, therapist, or pastor with whom to talk.

I can't stress strongly enough the importance of changing the negative attitudes and destructive behaviors currently in your life. Have you thought about the fact that you might become pregnant? It only takes once, you know. And what about sexually transmitted diseases such as gonorrhea and AIDS? Has your boyfriend had other sex partners? And have those sex partners had relationships with others? The nightmare grows and grows when you start to think about it.

You already know your behavior is unsafe and immature—you've said as much in your letter. *So stop it!* If you were running into fast-moving traffic for the fun of it, you could stop that behavior. You can also stop this one.

My mom is angry with me because she found me alone with my boyfriend in his apartment. If they forbid me to see him, I'll rebel and make their lives a living hell. I won't let them tear us apart. They say he's a fast, smooth-talker who might talk me into doing something I don't want to do. They don't know I've already been in a sexual situation with him, and that he didn't do anything I didn't want him to do. I had a boyfriend who tried to rape me in the backseat of his car. I think the reason why I can't let myself have sex now is because whenever I'm at the point of intercourse, everything that happened with my old boyfriend comes back to haunt me. I get all tight and remember the fear I felt with him. I'm still a virgin, but I don't want to be. I don't think I'll ever get over my fear of sex, and I'll end up being a virgin for the rest of my life. I'm so confused.

—Em

Your virginity is a gift that you can only give once. I realize this might sound corny to many teenagers, but it is true. How wonderful it is if you can give the gift of your virginity to your husband on your wedding night. What a marvelous act of love. Think about this before you seek to give away the most personal, private part of you.

Sex after marriage is God's plan and it works for several reasons. If you save yourself for your husband (or wife), you will have no regrets and no remorse. There will be no wishing that you could go back and undo mistakes you've made. Your self-respect will remain intact. There will be no loss of self-esteem (no feeling dumb, stupid, or used). (It's rather sad, isn't it, if all you have to offer the man you love enough to marry is "used goods"?)

Imagine your virginity as a wonderful gift for your husband on your wedding night.

God sees your body as a temple. You should too. All this doesn't mean that sexual intercourse is always wrong. The negative experiences you've had *can* be overcome with a patient, gentle, understanding husband.

It makes me sad when teenagers see themselves as being "at odds" or even "at war" with their parents. Please know this—*Your parents love you. They want the very best for you. They are only trying to protect you. Give them a chance!*

This is especially true in the case of someone who has suffered a date rape. This is something you cannot get over by yourself. You need counseling. If you don't get it, this issue will haunt you for the rest of your life. It may tarnish the relationship you have with any other man. Don't go to another guy to prove to yourself that you can have sex. You were hurt emotionally even more than you were hurt physically. You need to find emotional healing in order to get on with your life. There are many counselors, therapists, and pastors who deal with such issues. Tell your parents what happened with your old boyfriend. Ask them to find someone you can talk to about this.

It seems that you really don't want this new boyfriend as badly as you want to prove to yourself that you can get over your fear of sex. Make getting your life straightened out your first priority. Once you have resolved your fear and anger, you may not even want to continue this relationship.

Remember, even though some really bad things have happened to you, you can always start fresh with God. He's there, offering you forgiveness and a fresh start in Him.

THIRTY-EIGHT

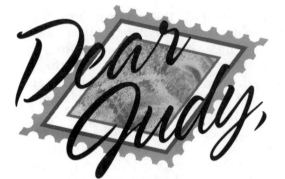

"My Friend Is Getting Too Serious With Her Boyfriend..."

● ● ● ● ● ● ● ● ●

I really need help. I'm living a story like the one in Book #5,
Broken Promises. *My friend Mia is going out with this boy,*
James. "Going out" at our school means being good friends and
holding hands, etc.

Three weeks ago, Mia invited James over without her parents'
permission. I felt guilty the whole night wondering what was hap-
pening and praying it would be all right.

I told my parents. I don't know if that was good or not, but I
was so worried that I knew it would slip out anyway. My friend
and I got into an argument and she accused me of telling my mom.
I told her I hadn't said anything to anyone. I know I shouldn't
have lied, but I had to or else I would have lost her as a friend.
She's still kind of mad at me.

—Niki, age 13

Your friend is angry with you because she knows what
she is doing is wrong and doesn't want to be caught at it.
Guilt is probably eating at her, but it is not painful or uncomfortable enough for her to stop her current behavior.

You've done what you can. It's too much for her to expect that you wouldn't talk to your mother about something that is troubling you so deeply. Now you must let this problem go. You cannot live your friend's life for her.

You can tell her what you think of her behavior and encourage her to really consider what she's doing. Maybe you can even hand her some of the pages of this book—the ones that apply to this situation. After that, all you can do is be there for her. (I wouldn't recommend lying again. Heaping lies upon lies doesn't solve any problem.)

There are some tactics that might make this discussion run a little more smoothly. Speak gently, not in a critical, harsh, or lecturing tone. *Plan* what you will say in advance so that you don't get caught up in the emotion of the moment and blurt out things you might later regret. Try to be compassionate and understand where your friend is coming from. See her side of the argument. Don't discuss this in the hallway at school. Pick a quiet time and place so that you can both be open, honest, and not frazzled.

If you feel you should do more (like talk to your friend's parents), I'd recommend that you discuss everything with your mom first. She can guide you.

I really like your books. Lexi and her friends have helped me through some rough times. They have also helped me learn some important things like:

Don't go too far with your boyfriend. I learned that in Broken Promises, *because Peggy and Chad went too far and Peggy got pregnant. That was a stupid thing to do. No girl would be dumb enough to have sex with her boyfriend.*

—Samantha

Ahhh . . . but lots of girls *do* have sex with their boyfriends. It is unfortunate but true. When you allow yourself to be ruled by emotion and passion, you will often do things you might regret later. Girls who have sex with their boyfriends are thinking of lots of things—but certainly not about their futures.

The best way to avoid trouble is to stay out of situations

that might be tempting. That means going out in groups more often and less single-couple dating. Lean on your parents for support in your dating relationship. Stick to social situations—restaurants, bowling alleys, mini-golf. And stay away (*far* away) from alcohol and drugs.

Dating relationships thrive in the sunlight. When the lights go out, the situation can quickly become uncomfortable and frightening.

Always remember that your body is *your* body. You don't have to share it with anyone. You have the right to say no. You have the right to put a stop to behavior that makes you feel uncomfortable. Respect your body. Respect yourself. You are a God-made, unique, beautiful treasure.

I have a real problem. My friend acts just like Peggy did in your book Broken Promises. *She kisses and hangs on her boyfriend in the halls at school. She* isn't *pregnant but she is getting closer to it. I know I should tell my parents, but if they call her parents I'll lose a friend.*

—Cloris, sixth grade

Have you talked to your friend? Have you told her that you're worried about her? Express your feelings, but do so gently. Also tell her how much you care about her and that you don't want to see her hurt. Explain that you see her and her boyfriend growing too close too fast.

Talk to your mom. Tell her what's troubling you. She knows your friend personally. Perhaps she can offer suggestions as to how to handle the situation. It's no fun to be alone with a problem. That's part of why God gave you parents. Take advantage of that gift!

It is important to realize that if you have this conversation with your friend, your fear might come true. You *may* lose a friend. It is difficult for a person to hear negative things about the choices they have made. But always do what you feel is best for your friends; in the end they may thank you.

THIRTY-NINE

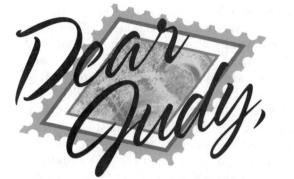

"My Best Friend Is Pregnant..."

• • • • • • • • •

This is the worst problem I've ever had. You have to help me! My friend is pregnant! She looks and acts exactly like Peggy Madison! My whole life is turning into a book!

I don't understand, Judy. I just don't. The baby is coming in five months. She already has morning sickness! She is excited about this but I'm not. I'm confused. I know she's confused too, more than she will admit. She's only thirteen. How could she do this? How could she! I'm scared, Judy. I'm really scared. I'm so scared, it's like I'm the one having the baby. I can't concentrate on schoolwork or anything! Help me! I need your answers as soon as I can or I'll die of worry and fear!

—Misty, age 12

You are upset because you are identifying closely with your friend. You've realized that if this could happen to your friend, it could happen to you. (If you made the same choices she did, that is.) You are imagining yourself in her position and it is terrifying you.

You can't change what has happened to your friend.

All you can do is trust that her parents and her doctor will see her safely through this pregnancy. And you can pray for her. Prayers are funny things, sometimes. You say prayers, giving them up to God, trusting that He will answer them. Sometimes you don't see quick results. After all, praying isn't like talking to the monitor at the drive-up window of a fast-food restaurant. You can't put your order in at one end and have someone hand it out a window at the other. You have to let God process the order in His own way. When you pray for your friend, ask God to help her through this time. God will know the best way to do that. Perhaps it will be by making her more calm and brave than she otherwise might be. Maybe He will give her strength or patience or good health (or all three). Pray for her and then trust God to answer in His own way and time.

There *are* a few things you can do for yourself. It appears that you are in a real tizzy over this situation and that you need to straighten out your own head.

First of all, try to understand why this happened. What behavior led your friend to this point? Rebellion? Loneliness? Experimentation?

Second, make the decision to never let this happen to you. Decide not to have premarital sex. It's as simple as that. Make the decision and carry through with it by not getting yourself in situations that could lead to trouble.

You may need to talk to someone who can calm you down. Talk to your mom and dad first. If you still don't feel better, go to your pastor or school counselor.

A freshman girl in our school had a baby last month. She did the same thing Peggy did in Book 5. She went to her friends and sister for help. She was going to have an abortion, then decided against it just like Peggy in Broken Promises. *She is back in school now. She has a baby-sitter and she's making up her school-work. You have opened my eyes!!*

—Celeste

Teen pregnancy is an eye-opener for all of us. We'd all like to pretend it's not happening, but, sadly, it is.

Make decisions early about the direction you would like your life to take. Set your goals high. Work to attain those goals. Don't jeopardize the future by taking detours (like alcohol or drugs) or dead-ends (like premarital sexual activity). Boys and sex may seem exciting and interesting now—and they are—but it's far better when the time is right.

The book Broken Promises *made me cry! When Peggy got pregnant, it made me wonder how old she is. I know a girl named Gail, who is seventeen and is pregnant. Is that bad?*

—Meredith

It certainly isn't good. An unmarried seventeen-year-old is going to have a tough time going to school, providing for and raising a baby. Her pregnancy has forced her onto a different path and it isn't an easy one. If she is planning to keep the baby rather than give it up for adoption, she now has some very difficult questions to face.

- How will she finish school?
- Will she have to go to work?
- How will she function during the day if she's been up all night with her child?
- Who will care for her baby during the day?
- Who will pay the bills—medical, food, baby clothes, sitters?
- Will she marry the baby's father? Is he old enough and mature enough to support her and the baby?

These questions only scratch the surface, but you get the picture. A baby changes *everything*.

Even if she gives the baby up for adoption, there will still be emotional problems to face. It's not easy to give up a child you've carried in your body for nine months. What's more, there will still be some physical reminders that she is a mother—sore breasts, stretch marks, etc.

Teenage sex can also be a *life and death* issue because of sexually transmitted diseases.

Is being seventeen and pregnant bad?

Sex is more than fun and games. Sex is the vehicle by which two people bring new life into the world.

At best it will be very difficult. You decide. It will change the life of the pregnant girl forever. God gave us rules to live by so that if we obey them, we will be safe from some of life's difficult situations. Learn a lesson from this girl. There's no need for you to make the same mistakes.

I had a friend get pregnant. Later she had an abortion.

—Deandra

One of my favorite passages in the Bible is Psalm 139. It talks about the fact that God knows everything. He knows all about us—when we sit down or stand up, what we think (before we even think it!), and every word we are going to say (before we even open our mouths!).

The Psalm goes on to say, "You [God] made my whole being. You formed me in my mother's body . . . You saw my bones being formed as I took shape in my mother's body . . . All the days planned for me were written in your book before I was one day old."

Abortion is not a method of birth control. It is a decision you must carry for the rest of your life.

It is interesting to think about this—to imagine God having a personal hand in the creation of each child who is to be born. It should certainly make each of us feel special. What's more, it should encourage us to reflect on the value of each individual life.

FORTY

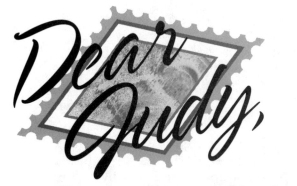

"My Boyfriend Abuses and Threatens Me..."

● ● ● ● ● ● ● ● ●

For the past three years I have dated John. He is a football player and very large. He is physically and mentally abusive to me. My life is similar to Peggy's in Something Old, Something New. *Every time I try to break up with him he says he will kill himself. Then he beats me up and tells me he will kill* me *if I don't stay with him.*

We haven't been dating lately, but for some reason, I still call him. I want him back, even knowing that he'll just put me down again. He'll come back, be nice for a while, and then accuse me of looking at some guy on the street. Then he'll yell at me, take me somewhere, hit me a few times, and get mad because I won't have sex with him.

Why is this happening to me? I was so nice to him! I forgave him for all his lies and all the girls he dated behind my back. He tells me I'm the best girl friend he's ever had. Why can't he treat me nicely? I give him everything he wants.

I know I shouldn't put up with his behavior, but I feel as though he has a hold on me. I don't really love him anymore, but he runs me down and makes me feel like I can't get anyone to love me. I am trying to fight back, but I don't think I have the mental strength to do it.

I have tried to get help from my parents and family, but they don't really know what to do or how to help.

Please help me. Sometimes I feel like I would be better off dead.

—Catherine, age 17

Get out of this relationship as quickly as you can and don't look back. No one, absolutely *no one*, has the right to abuse you. Your "boyfriend" (though he is hardly a friend) is mentally ill. He needs help. You must protect yourself. You are too deeply embroiled in this situation to see how sick it really is.

He is controlling you by ruining your self-esteem. He is making you believe that you have no value to anyone other than himself or that no one else could love you. This is absolutely *false*! Please don't believe his lies.

You *are* lovable! "You were bought with the precious blood of the death of Christ, who was like a pure and perfect lamb" (1 Peter 1:18–19). You *are* loved. You are one of God's children. Don't let anyone diminish that wonderful fact.

What's more, he is manipulating you by telling you that he will kill himself if you don't do as he says. That threat is the tool he uses to keep you in line and to make you do whatever he wants you to do. Frankly, there is as much danger that he will kill *you* when he is beating you as there is he will kill himself.

He does not own you. He is wrong to threaten and beat you. You must put a stop to it. *Do not call him again.* He will not change without professional help.

You must make the decision never to let him into your life again and then *do it*. If he calls you, don't talk to him. Avoid this boy. Protect yourself. If he hits you again, don't be afraid to call the police. It would even be wise to document any injuries with photographs. He is not only breaking your heart, he is breaking the law.

There are many wonderful, loving, considerate, gentle

men in this world. You don't need to keep going back to a cruel one.

You said you asked your parents for help—ask them again. Tell them you'd like to go to counseling. Tell them you need to learn how to handle this boy and how to handle your own feelings and insecurities.

If you are in an abusive situation, *get out as fast as you can*. Men who abuse won't change without professional help.

This boy has taken something very precious from you—your self-respect and self-esteem. Now it is time for you to reclaim it. It won't be easy. Though you may be tempted to call him, don't do it. Your life will be happier without *any* boyfriend than it is with this guy. You have the possibility of an exciting, marvelous life ahead of you. Look ahead to that, not back to what you've left behind.

You must find someone to talk to about your feelings (a counselor, doctor, or pastor). You must begin to heal. Remember that God is always nearby, always ready to listen. "Trust God all the time . . . tell Him all your problems. God is our protection" (Psalm 62:8). And He can do more for you than just listen because God promises to "heal the brokenhearted, and bind up their wounds" (Psalm 147:3). He's the One who can help you to feel better about yourself and get on with your life. Trust His promises. You can get through this.

My friend was being sexually harassed by an acquaintance. Reading your book Fill My Empty Heart *helped us make the right choices concerning her problem. We told her family and she is getting help. I would like to say that we owe it to your book.*

—April

That's good news! It is difficult and frightening to experience harassment and not know where to turn. My first recommendation is always to go to your family. If that doesn't work out, go to a teacher, a pastor, a neighbor, a doctor—anyone you feel close to who might help you. Sexual harassment among high school and even grade school students is not uncommon. Some schools have begun to formulate policies to deal with such complaints.

If the first person you approach is unwilling or unable to help you, don't give up. Go to someone else. Whoever is harassing you should be stopped.

FORTY-ONE

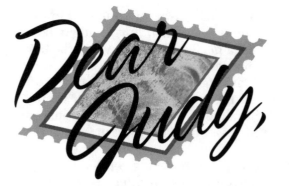

Just a Thought About Boys...

● ● ● ● ● ● ● ● ●

Last year I had a lot of problems with my friends and boys, but this year it has been totally different. I'm not tied down with a boyfriend and I feel great. I'm getting to do the things I enjoy most—cheerleading and gymnastics.

—Tawny

Good for you! You've learned an important lesson—one that not every teenager figures out. As you've read in earlier portions of this book, many (or most) girls (some as young as fifth or sixth grade) are so eager to have boyfriends that they convince themselves that their lives simply aren't interesting or fulfilled without them! They don't believe that they are whole or complete unless there is a boyfriend somewhere in their lives.

You, however, have come through that stage to the other side and realized that life *can* be just as exciting and fulfilling *without* a boyfriend as with one! You've taken one more step toward becoming an independent, mature, self-confident adult.

I don't want to bad-mouth boys, of course, (I think they're one of God's finest creations), but having a boy-friend doesn't guarantee a perfect life. Even when the boy you date is practically flawless, there is a downside.

If your boyfriend is around the house all the time, you probably won't have all the study time you need or the privacy you'd like. What's more, when you devote time to a boyfriend, you take hours *away* from others in your life—girlfriends, family, etc.

A steady boyfriend tends to make a girl too focused—on him. She may not have the time or interest to explore what is really most important for a teenager to investi-gate—personal interests, hobbies, sports, music, career fields. High school is a time to discover who you are as a person, not to pair up like the animals on Noah's Ark.

You have made a great discovery. *You* are the person with whom you have to spend the rest of your life. Learn to know yourself. Learn to be happy and content when you are alone as well as with friends. Discover the value and importance of *you*. Then you will become a marvelous life-partner for whomever you eventually marry.

PART III

Faith and Friends

● ● ● ● ● ● ● ●

*You will be my witnesses . . . in every
part of the world.*

Acts 1:8b

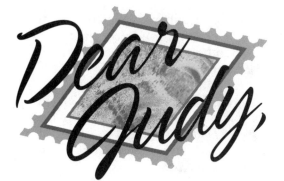

FORTY-TWO

"Do I Dare Let My Friends Know I'm a Christian?"

●　●　●　●　●　●　●　●　●

Lexi is a person I want to be like. I go to a public school too. Lexi wants everyone to know about her Christianity, but that's hard to do when you want your friends to accept you. I hear a lot of bad language at school. I do things I don't want to do, but I'm afraid my friends won't like me if I don't do them. How can I improve?

—Stacey

Do you like *yourself* if you do things you really don't want to do? That is the important question. You'd better make up your mind on which side of an issue you want to stand—and then stay there!

You don't have to make a big deal of things to get your point across. When someone asks or expects you to do something that you don't want to do, just say, "No thanks. I don't want to." You don't have to be judgmental or preachy. Be firm and pleasant. Who knows? There may be others who don't want to go along with the crowd either—be a leader for them, a role model.

Besides, if you are a Christian and are trying to follow

God's laws, then you've got an ally in your corner—the Holy Spirit. The Holy Spirit can let you know what to say, how much to say, and when best to say it in order to help others know Jesus. Ask Him to help you out.

Sometimes I feel so confused. It is so hard to act Christian-like during school. I hope you can give me a tip or two. How can I stay faithful to our heavenly Father? During school I get made fun of and criticized. I try to talk to my mom but she doesn't understand! There is nobody I can talk to!

—Molly, age 12

What exactly is "Christian-like"? It sounds like a "holier than you" attitude that would drive people away.

Being a Christian means having a personal relationship with Jesus Christ and accepting His death on the cross as a personal sacrifice He made for you. It also means that because of this amazing, loving gift, you want in return to be the best, nicest, most conscientious, and even happiest person you can be. Why? Because you know that God loves you, that Jesus died for you, and that your future in heaven is assured because of all that love. Why wouldn't you want to show your own gratitude and love for this gift by reciprocating with all the enthusiasm you can muster?

Christianity isn't a behavior that you put on like a jacket. It is *part of who you are.*

Christianity is an attitude, a *faith*, that is part of who you are—just as your blood and bones are part of your body.

Now, what is it that inspires the teasing and the criticism? Think about it. Ask yourself what you could do differently that would not bring such negative responses. (I'm not saying this is all your fault. I just want you to analyze the situation and see if there is anything you can do to improve it.)

Sometimes people who have recently received Christ into their lives get so enthusiastic about the event that they go too far with their enthusiasm. People who haven't yet experienced Christ's love in their own lives can be skittish about this overwhelming enthusiasm. Occasionally we do the exact opposite of what we hope to do. We mean to tell others how great a relationship with God can be, and instead we go too far too fast and scare them away.

That doesn't mean you should keep quiet about your beliefs. Ask the Holy Spirit to guide you in this matter. He'll show you what to say and how to act.

Like Lexi, I didn't want to compromise my beliefs for my friendships. That meant I often found myself alone. After taking the time to really find myself and to strengthen my relationship with God, I found friends who shared my beliefs or cared enough to respect them. I feel like you wrote Cedar River Daydreams books for me to encourage me in my own Christian walk!

—Monica, age 16

Your books have really helped me! I'm a Christian girl in the seventh grade. Your books and characters are a lot like me. We have the same problems! People at school make fun of me when I tell them I'm a Christian, 'cause they think Christians can't have a life!

—Mona

And they are so wrong! A Christian's life can be the most full (and fulfilling) of all.

It is very hard to be a teenager and a Christian at the same time.

—Julie, age 14

True. Very true. You do have some help for this, however. Here are a few samples.

"Be strong and brave and wait for the Lord's help" (Psalm 27:14).

"The Lord loves justice. He will not leave those who worship him. He will always protect them . . ." (Psalm 37:28).

Feel better?

FORTY-THREE

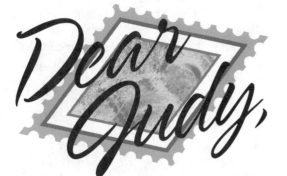

"How Do I Tell My Friends About Jesus?"

• • • • • • • •

One of my closest friends doesn't believe in God. She's the type that needs proof for everything and has to see things for herself. I've tried talking to her about it, but she's so strong-willed that she won't listen to me. I wish she'd stop making fun of God and invite Him into her life. I know she'd be so much happier. What should I do?

—Shelly

I recently moved, just like Lexi in New Girl In Town. *I have problems fitting in. My only real friends don't go to church or believe in God. How can I help them?*

—Jamie

First of all, there's no way you can argue or talk your friend into believing. In 1 Peter 3:15–16 it says, "Always be ready to answer everyone who asks you to explain about the hope you have. But answer in a gentle way and with respect. . . . Then those who speak evil of your good life in Christ will be made ashamed." That means you must always respond to your friend's negativity with love and patience.

You say your friend is strong-willed and won't listen to you. How about *showing* her what you believe? Introduce your friend to the Christian life by being the "light"—showing Christ's way through your actions. Make your friend wish she, too, had your calmness, your kindness, your compassion. You can talk until you are blue in the face, but if your actions say something else, you can't be a good witness.

That's what witnessing is all about—living your life in a special and appealing manner that makes others take notice.

Ask your pastor or youth group leader for other ideas. Is there an exciting event coming up—a Christian rock concert? a camp-out? anything you know that would interest even your doubting friends? Include them. Prove to them that Christians can have fun too.

You have the opportunity to introduce someone to Christ—that's exciting. But you do need Christian friends as well, to build you up if things go wrong, to remind you of what are the really important things in life.

It's a difficult tightrope we walk sometimes, being *in* this world but not *of* this world. We are citizens of this planet. This is where we exist. Yet, because of our belief in Christ, we function under a slightly different set of rules from those who do not share our beliefs. We're here. We have to be the best possible citizens of the world that we can be—and yet we have to remember that our first loyalty is to Christ and His commands.

This year I'm going to a public junior high school. Last year I went to a Christian school. I'll be in eighth grade. I am a little scared! When I went to a public school before, I wasn't the greatest Christian example. I gave my parents a rough time. I'm not proud of that! When I go back to public school, I'll be seeing a lot of people that I knew before when I was acting pretty dumb. This year I'll have to change the way they think of me. I've asked God to give me strength. It isn't going to be easy to start over.

—Elise, eighth grade

Dear Judy,

One of the marvelous things about God is that He not only *forgives* He *forgets*. Your classmates might not be quite so generous, but I have a hunch they'll give you a chance.

It is important that from now on you be *consistent* in your behavior. Those classmates will be watching you, and they will catch you if you stumble. Perhaps that's not all bad. Use it as a reminder that you've changed, that you are someone new now that you know Christ. Your attitude is good. You will make it.

I'm a Christian with a strong faith, but I've always been afraid that if people found out about my beliefs, they would hate me. Lexi and her friends have shown me that I should not be afraid. Thanks a lot.

—Laurie, age 12

I'm glad you're learning to be comfortable with your faith. Just remember that there are lots of ways to let people know that you are "different" than they are and that actions *do* speak louder than words. If you are consistently kind, courteous, cheerful, tolerant, etc. you'll stand out in a crowd. Just mentioning that you enjoy attending church or that you are a Christian will provide others with the opportunity to "put two and two together." They'll figure out that *who* you are has something to do with *what you believe*.

Also, not everyone is equally comfortable talking about the issue of personal faith. Perhaps you can discuss it one on one, but don't like to talk about it in a big crowd. That's okay. Know yourself and your limits and don't push yourself beyond what you are comfortable with and capable of at the moment.

This is a growing process. And just like you can't force a little boy to grow a beard and learn to drive until he is physically ready, you shouldn't expect to talk and act like a theologian or a pastor when you first begin to express your beliefs. Calm down and do what comes naturally. God will help you with the rest.

FORTY-FOUR

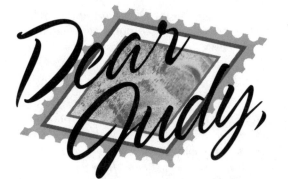

"I Get Embarrassed When I Talk About God . . ."

●●●●●●●●

I don't understand how Lexi can talk so freely about God. I'm a Christian and have been for a long time. I always get embarrassed when I start talking about God. Could you explain?

—Sheridan, age 11

I find myself ashamed to talk about my religion or beliefs. I feel badly about this and am trying to change. I go to a Christian school, but it's still hard to do what's right and to discuss God with friends.

—Gretchen, age 15

Lexi really had guts to talk to Matt about the Lord. I know that I never would have talked to Matt because he would say that I was pressuring him and that he doesn't believe in God. That book really touched my heart. I know how Matt would feel in real life because my parents are divorced and my mom is remarried. I have a hard time understanding my stepfather.

—Harmony

Dear Judy,

Why is it harder to witness to your neighbors than to complete strangers? Neighbors and strangers will both judge you, but you have to face your neighbors every day—I think that's why it's so tough.

—Rosemary, sophomore

Sometimes it is so hard! (Life I mean!) Sometimes, I think that instead of being a Christian, I'd prefer kissing a cow! I hide what I really am because I don't want to embarrass myself. Now I don't know who I am! Who is the real me? I just can't figure it out!

—Payton, age 13

I love reading Cedar River Daydreams *because they are so up-to-date on a teenager's life. Lexi helped me to realize that it is okay to share my feelings about religion with my friends and not feel embarrassed about it.*

—Heather, age 13

As a Christian and a teenager, it is hard to preach to your friends. But Lexi tells her friends and the people around her about her faith in God in a simple way. Ever since I have been reading your books, I've been more open about my feelings toward God.

—Diane

I have a hard time talking about God's word to my friends.

—Elaine

I find myself wishing I had the guts Lexi does to talk to people about Jesus.

—Juliana

I think Lexi is really brave!!!

—Sherry

I've written to you once before and I mentioned a problem of mine: I don't have any saved friends.

—Greta

I wish so much that I could be like Lexi when she witnesses to people. When I try (which is, truthfully, not often) I don't do very well. Do you know how I could improve?

—Ramona, age 14

Your books have shown me that knowing God is not something to hide. When you are proud of it, you can help others come to know Him also.

—Shirley

I like the way Lexi is able to witness so discreetly. She just brings it up and now she's even gotten Minda interested.

—Sheryl

This is a common problem for young Christians. It's not always easy for older Christians either. It is difficult (or perhaps the more accurate word is *emotional*) to talk about something that you feel so deeply and believe and value so much. This is a subject close to your heart. Understand that it's not abnormal to feel hesitant. In fact, it gets easier with practice. Do what you are comfortable doing. Ask the Holy Spirit for the words to say, the timing, the wisdom, and the bravery to accomplish your task. Relax. Then, when the time is right, you will know it. That may sound a bit strange to you, but it is true. If you have asked God for help and are truly listening for His answer, then you will know when it comes. (It's a little like God giving you a mental shove when you need it most!)

Don't underestimate the power of just a few comments when God is behind them.

And remember—you don't have to be a famous preacher to get your message across. Sometimes a few appropriate words are much more effective than a lengthy lecture about faith.

Dear Judy,

You are the holders of good news, *great* news, life-altering news! Christ loved us so much that He died for us. If He did that, He can certainly give you the appropriate words for every situation. Count on it. Count on Him.

FORTY-FIVE

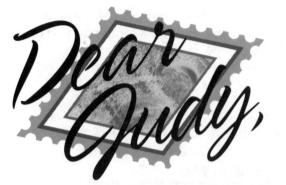

"I Feel as if I'm the Only Christian Around . . ."

● ● ● ● ● ● ● ● ●

Sometimes I feel like I'm the only kid in the world who really loves Jesus and wants to know Him better.

—Sandy, age 12

One of my problems is that I don't have many friends. The friends I do have are unsaved.

—Priscilla

Sometimes faith can be a lonely venture—but there really are many others who love Jesus and want to know Him better. This book proves that.

Perhaps you are looking in the wrong places for support. What's happening at your church? Youth group? Bible study? Sometimes (at least in the community I live in) youth groups invite people from other churches to share in activities. Ask your mom or pastor to help you explore the possibilities.

Are there people in your church you don't know?

Someone your age? Introduce yourself. Make a new friend. Who knows, maybe she's been hoping to meet someone just like you.

Bible camp is a great way to meet people with interests similar to yours. Have your mom go to the church office and check it out.

Unfortunately, friends don't just fall out of the sky. It takes both time and opportunity to develop friendships.

Fortunately, finding friends is something that you can leave in God's hands. He knows what you need—ask Him to help you find the right friends. (God doesn't mind. He likes to be involved in *every* aspect of your life—let Him.)

FORTY-SIX

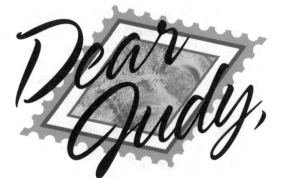

"People Think I'm a Loser Because I'm a Christian..."

● ● ● ● ● ● ● ● ●

I have a problem. Everybody thinks I'm a loser because I'm a Christian. Could you help me?

—Miranda

Here's a Bible verse that might give you some encouragement:

"When people insult you because you follow Christ, then you are blessed. You are blessed because the glorious Spirit, the Spirit of God, is with you. . . . If you suffer because you are a Christian, then do not be ashamed" (1 Peter 4:14, 16).

In other words, this sort of tormenting, teasing, and being told you are a loser if you follow Christ has been going on for a long, *long* time.

This doesn't mean, however, that *all* the suffering in your life is a result of your commitment to Christ or that this gives you permission to groan and moan that people always pick on you because of your beliefs. You also have to examine your behavior to make sure that you aren't inviting problems because of your own negative actions or attitudes. Have you ever heard someone complain that they aren't popular because they're a Christian, when you know, in fact, that their unpopularity has much more to do with a crummy attitude or an unpleasant personality? A painfully honest self-examination once in a while should keep this particular problem from occurring.

What this verse *does* promise is that Christ will be there for us *totally* whenever we stand up for Him. He's in our court, behind us 100%. Good news, right?

When you were in junior high, did kids ever tease you about being a Christian or not knowing any of the rock songs they do? I'm having trouble with that at school this year. I don't understand why people do that! Do you know how I could stop them from bothering me?

—Mitzi

While you are growing up, teasing is inevitable. Kids like to pick on anyone who is different from the "norm" or from themselves. Because you aren't familiar with certain things (such as rock lyrics), you are a bit out of step with your classmates and an easy target for teasing.

First of all, how *do* you respond?

Do you get mad? Cry? Lash out? Try to defend yourself?

Instead of whatever it is you do, try something different for a while. If you usually get teary-eyed or angry, try to smile and shrug it off.

A clever or savvy response may be the best way to diffuse the teasing. Plan in advance what you might say when this situation develops.

Another idea might be to simply not respond at all to the teasing. Let it wash over you and ignore it. Make yourself a poor target. Don't be fun to tease anymore!

If it gets really bad you might try talking to your teacher about this. Maybe he or she will have a suggestion for you.

Avoid those who tease you. Find the friends who respect your beliefs and try not to worry about the others. It's hard, but there's no easy way to make intolerance go away.

Don't be discouraged. Christ accepts you and He's the One who really counts! One or two of your tormentors may eventually get the picture and begin to wonder what they are missing in their own lives.

It is hard being a Christian. That's why I like reading about Lexi. She's my role model. I want to be like her. She is such a strong Christian, and she has lots of Christian friends. I don't have a whole lot of big problems, but it is nice to know being a good Christian can be done. Sometimes I need that boost. My biggest problem is witnessing. Is inviting someone to church witnessing? If it is, then maybe I have witnessed.

—Vanna

Yep. That's one way—and it wasn't so hard, was it? I think people should do whatever is comfortable for them. Once inviting friends to church with you comes easily, you may find yourself wanting to do more. Great. Do it. We have to give ourselves permission to be who we are. Some people are excellent witnesses through their words. Others shine through their actions. A few (like me) do it through their writing. God didn't make us all exactly the same. He doesn't expect us to behave exactly the same either.

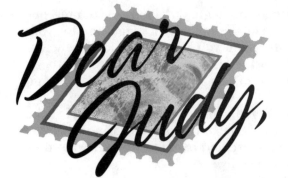

FORTY-SEVEN

"My Friends Tease Me About Being a Christian..."

●●●●●●●●●

I'm always trying to serve God. That's the problem. Because of that I'm considered a "goody-goody." I don't fit in at all. I'll start high school in a couple of weeks and I'm scared to death! I want friends so badly, but I don't feel comfortable with kids who aren't Christians. Can you help me? I've prayed but I'm sort of on hold.

—Ronnie, age 14

It is great that you are trying to serve God. I wouldn't want to discourage you from doing that—but is there any chance that your attitude is contributing to your current problems?

Sometimes when people try so hard to do what is good and right, they get what is called a "holier-than-thou" attitude. You know what I mean. It's a really annoying manner that announces to the world (or the person you are talking to), "I don't smoke (or cheat at school, or gossip, etc.), and that makes me a better person than you are." It's an easy trap to be caught in.

Unfortunately it sometimes happens to Christians. When it occurs, it has the unhappy result of doing the exact *opposite* of what you really want (which is, of course, to draw others *to* Christ). You may desperately want to show others how wonderful it is to know Christ personally, but a holier-than-thou attitude may send them scurrying in the opposite direction instead.

Please don't worry so much about going to high school. Christ walked with non-Christians every day. He *came* to earth because of non-Christians.

Jesus' disciples were a real hodge-podge of people and lifestyles. Simon Peter showed his weak, human side many times. He and the other disciples said they would never desert Jesus. But, of course, when things got serious, that's exactly what Peter did—he denied that he knew Jesus.

Another of Jesus' disciples was doubting Thomas—he needed proof for everything before he would believe it. When the others told Thomas that Jesus had risen from the dead, Thomas said, "I will not believe it until I see the nail marks in his hands. And I will not believe until I put my finger where the nails were and put my hand into his side" (John 20:25). (See what a doubter he was?)

What does this tell us? That Jesus came for *all* of us. And He especially wants to get His message out to non-Christians. Who knows? Maybe He has a plan for you at this new high school. Only God knows that.

Christ walked with non-Christians every day. In fact, He came to earth for the non-Christians!

I'd recommend that you try to relax. You're allowing yourself to become all stressed out. Instead, ask God to help you in this new environment. If you really want to serve God, then you should ask Him to help you do just that.

Your books have made me realize that I am not as good a Christian as I should be. Sometimes I can be a hypocrite. That is something that I do not want to be. It is not easy being a Christian, even at a Christian school. You still get laughed at. My classmates laugh at me and my friends. I am a straight-A student and try not to get demrits. Most of my classmates think that I think I'm "Miss Perfect."

—Hannah, seventh grade

I don't have any Christian friends at school and I experience "peer pressure" every day! It is very hard for me. My friends all know I'm a Christian. I'm not what my pastor calls a "secret Christian." I get good grades in school and have a great family. Kids at school call me "Barbie doll." They say I'm perfect. What upsets me is that I am not perfect. I study forever to get good grades. I guess there are worse things to be called than "Barbie," but it still bothers me. From now on, whenever I'm in a bad situation I'm going to ask myself what would Lexi do if she were in my shoes?

—Roxanne, age 13

When you are really trying to do your best, occasionally other people will take perverse pleasure in pointing out how "different" you are. Instead of taking this as an insult, perhaps you should take it as a compliment.

You get good grades, have a great family, enjoy a strong spiritual life, and know Christ personally as your Savior. Which of those things would you give up in order to be more popular? *None,* I would guess. It seems to me that what you already have is *worth* tolerating a little hassling for. Realistically, you would never give up what you have to be more like your friends, so I'd recommend accepting the good with the bad (and there is definitely more good than bad in your life).

The only person you can change is yourself. Revamping your own attitude might be the most efficient way to deal with the problem.

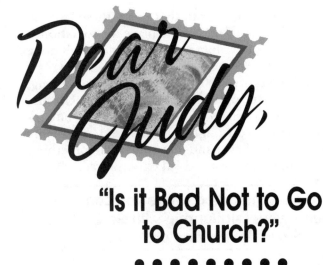

FORTY-EIGHT

"Is it Bad Not to Go to Church?"

● ● ● ● ● ● ● ● ●

Is it that bad not to go to church? My friend says it is. I don't see why it would be. Is being a really strict Christian bad?

—Monique

Is it bad just to eat high-calorie, high-fat junk food and never eat protein, fruits, or vegetables? In order for your body to grow and thrive, you need to nourish it properly and give it the nutrients that make healthy bones and strong muscles.

In order to thrive spiritually, you have to nourish yourself too—and church is one place to find that nourishment. You might not *die* if you lived your life eating only chips, salsa, and soda pop, but you wouldn't bloom and prosper either. The same thing goes for church and your spiritual life.

Not every minute of church is exciting, stimulating, or educational. Frankly, sometimes it can really drag. *But,* at the same time, something rather wonderful is happening. We are told of it in Matthew 18:20: "If two or three people come together in my name, I am there with them."

God is there! It's His house. It's the place we go to honor and worship Him, to say "Thanks, Lord!" for all He's done for us.

Church can't be taken lightly. Even if it seems boring, go anyway. Your attitude can make a difference. Use the time to talk to God, listen to the music, think of your relationship with Him. You might be surprised. The Holy Spirit can work in your heart and mind and turn something you think is boring into a wonderful experience.

Church is the place where you can nourish your relationship with God— keeping it vital and growing.

Here are some more ideas for making church a more meaningful experience:

1. Take *notes*. (It's a great way to make yourself pay attention to everything that's being said.)
2. Really *listen* to the pastor. (Sometimes you might even find yourself disagreeing with what he says. If that happens, ask yourself why you disagree. Think about what you believe. Jot down questions you'd like to ask the pastor later.)
3. *Relax* and let the music and prayers flow over you. (You'll be amazed how soothing and energizing that can be.)
4. *Invite* Jesus into your head and your heart. Savor the peace and joy you'll feel when He comes.

This guy in my class says that he doesn't believe in Jesus. He says that if Jesus existed He would save us from teachers, earthquakes, wars, fights, homework, and stuff like that. I said maybe it is because too many people have done wrong, and that might be a way to punish them.

He asked how we even know that there is a God. How do we know He is coming back? I hope you can give me some hints.

—Michalean, age 11

That's what faith is all about—believing what we cannot see. We do it on a smaller, less important level every day. I can't see electricity, yet I know it's humming through the wires of my house. I have faith it's there, and therefore I won't do something stupid like trying to blow-dry my hair in a bathtub full of water. I can't see germs or viruses floating in the air or on the dirty ground, yet I believe they are there and wash my hands before I eat a meal so I don't get sick. I'm writing this book on a computer that works even though I have absolutely *no* idea how! I have faith that if I press the keys, the letters will be imprinted, first on a disk, later on paper. Amazing, but it works.

Faith is about believing what we cannot see.

Jesus doesn't *cause* earthquakes. He doesn't send catastrophes of nature to kill hundreds of His children. A shifting of the earth's crust causes earthquakes. He doesn't cause war either. Human beings have to take credit for that. What He *does* do, however, is stand beside us when we need help to pick up the pieces and straighten out the messes we've made of our lives.

We live in an imperfect world. We have a free will. We like to make our own choices. When we make the wrong ones, He is there for us.

Jesus is real, all right. Your friend just hasn't met Him personally yet.

FORTY-NINE

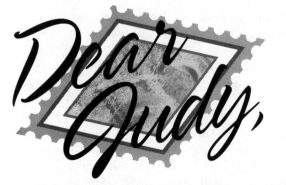

"Why Can't I Say I'm Sorry?"

● ● ● ● ● ● ● ● ●

If you're supposed to forgive others, why can't I bring myself to say "I'm sorry"?

—Matty

It's a one-word answer. Pride. You don't want to admit having made a mistake. It goes against everything in you to admit you goofed. Lots of people suffer with this problem—it's so common, in fact, that references to pride are sprinkled throughout the Bible.

"Pride will destroy a person. A proud attitude leads to ruin" (Proverbs 16:18).

It's not easy to admit your imperfections. Many people spend their lives trying to pretend they are perfect. There is nothing strange about admitting that you are human. It's comforting to know that everyone can goof up at one time or another.

When you can admit to making a mistake, people usually like you *more*, not less.

You may actually have to *practice* saying you are sorry. It doesn't always roll easily off the tongue—but it usually does feel better once you've said it.

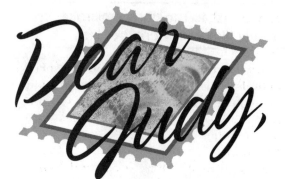

FIFTY

"Why Don't My Friends Take God Seriously?"

● ● ● ● ● ● ● ● ●

I belong to a Bible study group. I lead the group. They are all my friends, but they can't seem to get serious about the Lord and really pray to Him during our study. Many laugh and play games during opening and closing prayer. These are my best friends and I love them, but they don't seem to have a very strong commitment to the Lord.

Some are Christian girls, but others are confused and lost. I can't seem to guide them all in the right direction. We start high school next year. I want them to be saved and to have a strong Christian faith to get through our tough years ahead. Most won't share. They talk to each other when I'm reading Scripture. Am I going about things wrong? They all say they want to be there. But, what are they coming for? Help!

—Ellen

Your friends are probably coming to Bible study for fun, fellowship, conversation, and the opportunity to be part of a group. Obviously, none of them wants to be left out. They probably also really do want to learn something about the Bible.

Then, why don't they listen?

Most likely the answer lies in their immaturity. They are still a little uncomfortable with such a serious topic. Obviously, there are also different levels of interest in Bible study within the group. Some want to visit more than they want to study. If one person wants to visit, it's easy to draw others into a conversation.

What's more, it is very difficult for someone of the same age to lead and manage a group of their peers. You've taken on a big responsibility. Is there someone else who could teach with you? A college girl or boy? Your mom? An older friend?

Don't be too hard on yourself and don't be discouraged. You never know just what it is that might spark a new interest of commitment from one of your friends.

FIFTY-ONE

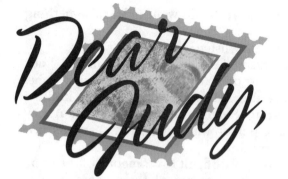

"My Friends Don't Act Like Christians..."

● ● ● ● ● ● ● ●

Some of my friends say *they are Christians, but don't act like it. They say bad words and listen to worldly music. They even skip school. I don't know what to say to them when they do that, but I want to tell them something.*

—Josie, sixth grade

I'm sure that is confusing to you, but it's a perfect example of what I mean when I say that actions speak louder than words. *Saying* you are a Christian but not *acting* like one sends mixed messages to the world.

If you want to discuss this with your friends, I'd recommend that you not take them all on at once. Wait for a good time when you are alone with just one friend. Gently tell her what's bothering you. Explain why you feel as you do. Remind her that you value her friendship and don't want this to come between you. Then trust God to work through your words. *You* can't do any more, but *He* can do marvelous things.

This is sad to say, but you may actually lose some of

your friends. They may not want to change. In fact, they may even want to drag you down too. I wish I had easy answers for everything, but I don't. But that's part of what life is about—making the best of the circumstances around us.

Saying you are a Christian but not acting like one sends mixed messages to the world.

My friend claims to be a Christian, but she lies and does other stuff like that. We used to be best friends, but now she likes my sister better than she likes me. I don't know why. Maybe I did or said something she doesn't like. Whenever I try to talk to her, she acts cold toward me. I always seem to make people mad at me, no matter how hard I try to be normal. I am so bothered about this because she is my only friend. Perhaps I have a massively rotten attitude that God is slow to change.

—Haley, age 13

Talk to your sister—perhaps she can give you some insight into your friend's attitude. If you discover that you've hurt her feelings, apologize. Tell her how much you value her friendship. That's all you can do. If she no longer chooses to be your friend, you cannot force her to do so. Then you must make new friends. As much as we would like to have everyone like us, it won't happen. It can't happen.

From your letter it appears that something else is also going on in your relationships with others. Reread these lines from the letter:

I always seem to make people mad at me, no matter how hard I try to be normal.

Something has gone wrong in your communication with others. In order to solve this part of the puzzle, you must look at both your attitude and your manner.

Dear Judy,

One of the most negative accusations I've heard my daughters make is, "He is so *annoying!*"

Are you sure you aren't being "annoying," even if you don't mean to be? When my daughters say "annoying," they mean irritating, snoopy, thoughtless, dorky, goofy, busybody-ish, or a dozen other aggravating things that drive them wild. Look at your own behavior just to make sure you aren't being annoying to those around you. If you catch yourself doing something that might irritate others, stop it. It's not easy to break habits, but it can be worth the effort. I'm sure there *is* someone out there who would be very happy to have a friend like you.

I actually thought I was making friends at church. I believed that until someone started acting strangely toward me. He told everyone that I was a stuck-up, conceited snob and that I think that I am better than everyone else. It may not sound like a big deal to you, but it hurts because now that is how everyone *sees me.*

I thought that born-again Christians were different from others, but they are not. They are like everyone else who hates me. I really thought that things would change and I'd actually have a true friend who would love me for who I am. Now all my friends have turned against me. I've managed to avoid church and fellowship for a while, but I can't avoid them anymore because my mom is becoming suspicious. I don't want my mom to know my personal life. She always blames me for everything and I'm not in the mood for one of her lectures.

What would you do if you were in my situation? What is there to do? Sometimes praying does not help at all! I know I should have more faith than that. I guess I am not supposed to be ashamed and upset over small things like that, but I am. For the first time in my life I am actually ashamed to show my face somewhere. The feeling is terrible. Even school is better than church!!!!!!!!

—Jolene

Talk to your mom. This is something you should not go through alone. Mom can be there for you; don't sell her short.

You may be mistaken that *everyone* sees you as a snob. It may only *feel* that way because you are hurting right now.

You may even need to talk to your pastor about this. He should know about a situation that drives someone—anyone—away from the church.

Church is not a place for the practically perfect. It is for people with weaknesses and flaws. It is also a place where *everyone* should feel welcome. Please don't let this situation drive you away.

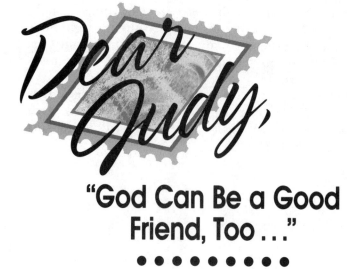

FIFTY-TWO

"God Can Be a Good Friend, Too..."

● ● ● ● ● ● ● ● ●

There are a couple of things that bother me a little about your books. One is the way you talk about God and praying. It is as though He is Lexi's good friend. Also, I wish you could make Todd and Lexi's relationship a little more serious. Other than that it is a great series. You cover all of the issues like teen pregnancies, feeling out of place, etc.

—Geena

He *is* Lexi's good friend! He's mine too. And He wants to be yours.

I have conversations with God in my mind all the time. I don't "save" some special, holy vocabulary for Him or wait until a certain hour to talk to Him. When I have a thought or a need, I tell Him! Look at what the Bible says about prayer:

"We can come to God with no doubts. This means that when we ask God for things (and those things agree with what God wants for us), then God cares about what we say. God listens to us every time we ask him. So we know that he gives us the things that we ask from him" (1 John 5:14–15).

"The Lord is close to everyone who prays to him, to all who truly pray to him" (Psalm 145:18).

Prayer is conversation with God. He loves you more than you can possibly imagine. He created you. You are His child.

You can talk to God just like you would talk to a good friend. He's listening.

It's very exciting to see Lexi get through tough times by prayer! I would love some tips on how to be more like her!

—Kathy

Be yourself! That's the best person you can be.

Lexi is always very aware of the spiritual aspects of her life. She practices what I call "applied Christianity." That means that with every aspect of her life she asks these questions: "What would Jesus want me to do or say in this situation? How would He want me to act? If Jesus were here, what would *He* do?"

If you keep that in your mind (and pretty soon it becomes second nature to you) you will be the best you can be.

Thanks a lot for your help. It really means a lot. Especially at my age, everything seems to go wrong.

—Jean

I hope this book has made you realize that you are not alone with your problems. From the questions you have read, you now know that *lots* of girls are having friend problems, boy problems, doubts, and fears.

There are two things that will make it easier to be a teenager. The first is *faith*. If you know God, you always have someone on your side (no matter what happens). You have a friend who will listen when others won't, and be there for you when others would leave.

The second is *attitude*. Only you can control how you feel about things and how you respond. If you can maintain a cheerful, upbeat, no-worries type attitude, things will go more smoothly for you. (Sometimes you have to pretend to be happy, but amazingly enough, if you act happy long enough you actually begin to feel that way!)

And to answer the question that formed the title for this book—Did I ever like a boy who didn't like me? Dozens of them. And there were boys who liked me even though I didn't like them! That's how life is.

One time I had a crush on a guy who didn't know I existed, and I thought my heart would explode in my chest.

Dear Judy,

He was so *cute*! And so *popular*! And so . . . sure never to be mine.

Not every boy is meant to like every girl in a romantic sense. That's okay. (Actually, you wouldn't even *want* them all to be crazy about you. What a problem it would be to sort out the true Mr. Right if everyone were after you!) Teenage years are great for trying out ideas, emotions, and experiences. Make the most of it and, please have fun!